RAFT

Also by Howard Goldenberg

My Father's Compass: A memoir

Raft

Howard Goldenberg

HYBRID
PUBLISHERS

Published by Hybrid Publishers
Melbourne Victoria Australia

©Howard Goldenberg 2009

First published 2009

National Library of Australia Cataloguing-in-Publication entry:
Author: Goldenberg, Howard 1947–
Title: Raft / Howard Goldenberg

ISBN: 9781876462857 (pbk.)

Subjects: Goldenberg, Howard
Aboriginal Australians – Social conditions – 21st century
Aboriginal Australians – Social life and customs
Aboriginal Australians – Health and hygiene

Dewey Number: 305.89915

Cover design: © Grant Gittus Graphics
Photos: © Brendan Finn
Painting on front cover: © Rod Moss – 'Raft' (1990)
Back cover photograph: © Brendan Finn – Author in front of 'Raft'

Typeset in Minion Pro 12/16.5
Printed in Australia by McPherson's Printing Group

The truth is rarely pure and never simple.

(Oscar Wilde, Algernon to Lady Bracknell in
The Importance of Being Earnest, Act I)

To Annette

CONTENTS

Places and Communities named in 'Raft'

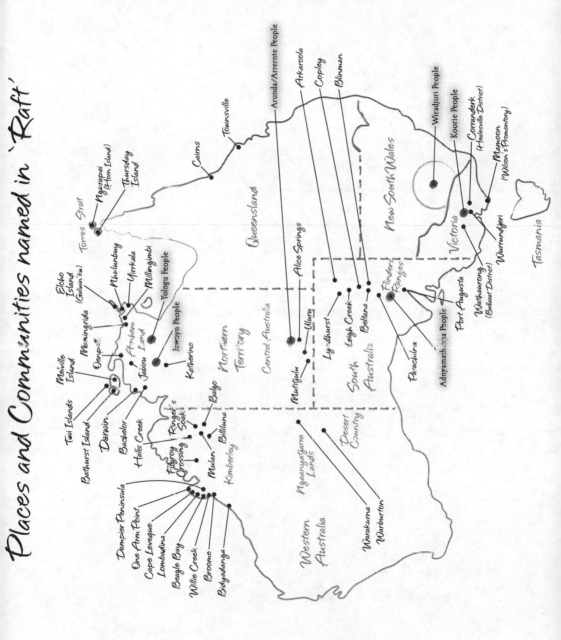

Ngurupai (Horn Island)
Thursday Island
Torres Strait
Cairns
Townsville
Queensland
Arunda/Arrernte People
Arkaroola
Copley
Blinman
Wiradjuri People
Koorie People
Corranderk (Healesville District)
Maroon (Wilson's Promontory)
New South Wales
Victoria
Warrnadjeri
Tasmania
Alice Springs
Flinders Ranges
Port Augusta
Wathaurong (Ballarat District)
Maningrida
Elcho Island (Galiwin'ku)
Nhulunbuy
Yirrkala
Milingimbi
Yolngu People
Arnhem Land
Larrakiya People
Oenpelli
Jabiru
Katherine
Northern Territory
Central Australia
Uluru
Ly- Whurst
Leigh Creek
Beltana
Adnyamathanha People
Parachilna
South Australia
NMartjitjalu
Twi Islands
Melville Island
Bathurst Island
Darwin
Batchelor
Halls Creek
Ringer's Soak
Fitzroy Crossing
Mulan
Balgo
Billiluna
Kimberley
Dampier Peninsula
One Arm Point
Cape Leveque
Lombadina
Beagle Bay
Willie Creek
Broome
Bidyadanga
Ngaanyatjarra Lands
Desert Country
Warakurna
Warburton
Western Australia

ix

PART ONE

RAFT

The emotions between the races could never be pure;
… the other race would always remain just that:
menacing, alien and apart.

(Barack Obama in *Dreams From My Father*)

1. THE RAFT

Thin legs

Riding my bike in the quiet dark, I make out two dark forms moving toward me. From near the top of one of the forms a red glow identifies the moving object as human. In Alice the glow of burning tobacco is one of the signs of the human condition, another being the sheen in the streetlight of the bottle of liquor. We are here in the Red Centre, the bleeding heart of Oz. Everywhere are the all-drinking all-smoking living lost, the people who are dying on the raft, or who have jumped from the raft, into this former inland sea.

Pedalling in the dark, I begin to make out the outline of the second human form. It follows closely behind the smoker, and moves, as he does, silently. The follower is of adult height and girth, but her legs are stick-figure thin, blackbirds' legs, mere linear props keeping the torso off the ground. The legs are, I realise immediately, too thin to be real. It must be the light, or the lack of light, playing a trick on my eyes; those black lines are ideas, insubstantial – even the bare tibial bones would be thicker than they. They could barely support, never carry forward that torso.

I draw alongside, and with the help of streetlight I can make out some detail. The smoker, like so many of the poor around these parts, is wearing the loose, formless trousers of the concentration camp victim. He is barefoot, about thirty-five, and steers his legs with difficulty. I have the impression of a gait which will not be better once the grog wears off, the gait not of intoxication but of some chronic damage.

The gait of the woman who follows mutely in his wake is, by contrast, steady and deliberate. She knows where she is going – she is going where she has to, where he leads her. She is, to judge from her face, beyond protesting.

And the legs, in this clearer light, are just as I first saw them, thin beyond belief. These are the legs of malnutrition. Only in the cachectic, in those dying of cancer, have I seen such legs. These are not the legs that would bear an Australian adult moving upon the soil of her country.

But of course, these people are black.

In the course of my first morning at work in Alice, I meet Gilbert and Beatrice and Samuel, all in their forties, all three dying already of premature age and despair; of alcohol, tobacco and neglect. These three radiate anger. The anger sears the hapless reception staff then it burns me in turn. The three were not born here. They do not know each other. They all came, fleeing the wreckage of their former lives, fleeing their problems, unaware that they were bringing their problems with them. They each took to the raft, unaware it was fatally overloaded.

Because they are white, they feel a right to their anger.

Of course there are able people, whole and hale, in Alice Springs. There are the tourists. They stroll the streets in rude good health and spirits – blondes from Northern Europe, Japanese, Scandinavians, Latins.

And there are the armies of public servants who heal, and teach, and rescue those on the raft. I am here to allow a healer a chance to have a holiday. I am a sort of rescuer for one of the rescuers.

An ancient mariner

A tall man with silver hair and brown skin enters my consulting room, hunched forward a little. His voice has the familiar huskiness of many of his people; his speech is deliberate.

'I cannot say quickly what is wrong, doctor. Please allow me time to explain.'

The face is a compound of care and charm. He is not young but he is well muscled and broad. He bends his torso somewhat, and inclines his head a little as he speaks, his mouth almost smiling – in propitiation? Has a lifetime among white people taught him to smile as he speaks, even when – as now – his speech is full of sorrow and care?

'I have a boy,' he says. 'He is twelve years old.'

Irresistibly, he begins to deliver his story. He needs no long grey beard, no glittering eye to arrest me. The consultation has stopped.

My patient continues, 'I've had him since he was a baby. He is my son's boy. The boy's mother brought him to me when he was newly born. She said – "You take this boy, I cannot look after him." I told her – "You need to think about that. You take him away and think again. A child needs his mother …"'

The man breaks off his narrative to explain his meaning. 'Doctor, I said that about a mother because I didn't have my mother with me when I was a boy. Well, she brought the baby back a couple of days later. She said, "You take this boy. I can't have him."'

A pause.

'Doctor, I've lost my licence to drive trucks. I want to get it back. I want to get back into work again. They say I can't drive trucks any more because of my heart and because I used to have diabetes. So I went to Adelaide and had heart tests. They put a needle into your groin and they send dye into your heart – you know?'

I nod.

'They tell me I am good, my heart is good. I feel good, doctor.

And when I came back, they tested me again, but they couldn't find any diabetes, because I am eating good food – you know – no Kentucky Fried … no Red Rooster. No grog either. I don't smoke. I am very strong, doctor, I am fit. Every morning and most nights I do hard exercise …'

I nod again, admiring his lean, muscled body.

'I am going to school. I am learning computer. That's hard, those words are very hard. I was raised on a Catholic mission in the Kimberley, out Fitzroy Crossing way. They didn't teach me much to read and write, not English. I learned mostly prayers … in Latin. I can still say all the prayers in Latin, but I don't understand Latin. I didn't have much schooling in the Kimberley.'

I look up and scan his face, looking for something that seems to be missing: where is the irony, where is the anger? He seems to have none.

'Last year my wife got sick. She was in the hospital, but in the end they say to me – "you take her". So I take her home. She was in the wheel chair, she liked to be outside. So I would take her out there, she'd sit in the chair with a mask on her face – for oxygen. The boy would come out to her and sit with her, and he would cry.

'I see them out there and I cannot bear it. I told the boy, "You have to go to your mother now. I can't look after you, you're too big for me now. You need your mother …" A boy needs his mother. I didn't have … The boy cried when I sent him back. He wanted to stop with me.

'My wife died. After a good while I went to my country, you know, the Kimberley, that's good country. I wanted to see my sisters …'

I contemplate the distance from where we sit, in Alice Springs. 'Did you fly?'

'I fly my car. I don't mind the drive, it is good country, beautiful, all the way. When I get there, the boy wants to be with me all the time. He camps with me, he won't stop with his mother.'

The man pauses, looks at me. The part-smile returns. 'Doctor, I need a letter so I can drive trucks again. I want to be working again. I have to do something …'

Heavily, I tell him that the doctor who decided he must not drive trucks is probably right. The law says a doctor can't let you drive trucks if you have a history of heart troubles. But I tell him I will obtain the reports from the Adelaide doctors and forward them to an independent heart doctor and see whether he can have another chance. I try not to raise his hopes.

The old man rises, takes my hand. The smile is full now, his hand large, dry, warm.

He thanks me and goes away. Sadder, wiser, I watch him go.

Business at the bank

Friday lunchtime, the bank is a sea of people, wave upon wave, waiting their turn to be served. There are three queues of customers treading water, waiting. One queue forms behind a sign that says something like: For people with the Patience of Job; another sign says: Form a Line Behind this Sign if You Cannot Read; and the last sign reads: Idiots Only. I step into this line, the shortest by a mile.

I notice that the first line is for middle-class people – the washed, the literate, the banking classes. In this line there are local white people, local black people and tourists. It is an orderly queue which inches forward.

The next line moves more slowly. It seems to be for Aborigines, generally out-of-towners. The line is a bit anarchic, the queuers are a bit skew-whiff, their apparel unconventional. Suddenly, one of them shouts something obscure and aggressive in a hoarse voice. He shouts again. No one answers, no one reacts. I look around to see whether Security will act to restore order, but Security is in fact busy outside the front, attending to an incident.

The incident in question has not yet actually taken place, but it appears as if it might at any moment. The incidental individual, a woman, has chosen to take a seat on the footpath immediately outside the bank, just next to the electric door. Through the plate glass windows Security can be seen approaching her, addressing her, apparently asking her to move on. She makes no response. And she does not move.

Security is a tall man in a very white uniform, with banana republic epaulettes. He holds a walkie-talkie. He again asks her to decamp. Nothing doing, so he speaks into his instrument, calling up reinforcements.

The reinforcement wears the same uniform. He is not so tall, but he has been to the gym, building up some muscle bulk to fill his uniform and gain a little respect from the public. The two officers in white bend over the woman. She does not move. She is a rock, a rock on the shore of the sea.

She is one, the officers are two. Things look a bit unequal to me. I look around at the treaders of water, and at the bank officers. No one seems to have noticed the woman outside. Apparently she is invisible, a condition quite common among black people in Alice Springs. She has not been seen by anyone inside, whether black or white.

I have been served quickly and courteously. Meanwhile, the woman remains marooned on the footpath. I step outside and observe the scene.

It is hot out here. Midday crowds pass in front, between and behind the three outside the bank, but no one sees the invisible one. Only Security and I can see her. I wonder why the invisible one makes no sound nor sign of awareness. Perhaps she is sick …

Suddenly I remember that I am a doctor. I bend forward and ask, 'Are you all right?'

No answer. I look at her minutely and am unable to decide whether she is at peace or at a loss. I cannot tell whether she sits here by choice or perforce; only the strength of her silence speaks.

Again I enquire, 'Are you sick?'

No response.

'Do you need help? Can I help you?' The woman stretches forth her right arm, half opening her hand, revealing a scrap of paper. She remains silent. What does she expect me to do – if anything? Gently, I flatten the paper in her palm and read its secret: '$318. Australia Post.'

This lady is poorly dressed. If this paper means that she owns – or is owed – $318, the sum is substantial, the fact is significant. Unfortunately, the fact is also profoundly obscure, as is everything about her. She clutches her little rectangle of paper like a talisman or a passport, but there is no one here to honour it.

As I retreat in confusion, I look back over my shoulder at the two security officers. They look just as confused as I feel. And the woman remains as she was, obdurate and oracular, a rock in a sea of unknowing.

◉◉◉

'Raft' is an important painting by Rod Moss of life and wreckage upon our own shores. It recalls Gericault's 'Raft of the Medusa', a work which depicts some of the survivors of the Medusa, the flagship of the French fleet, whose loss in fine weather was felt by the French to be both a scandal and a national shame. Gericault's painting shows the survivors who took to a raft. Their desperate postures and the eerie green tinge of their flesh cry out in an agony of degradation and hopelessness.

Rod Moss painted his own 'Raft', showing indigenous figures marooned in the landscape. Those capable of standing search a distant horizon for a rescuer; one points to something that is not seen. Over the whole scene, there is a palpable silence.

Central to the scene is a woman, not young, probably wife and mother to the wrecked. In a scene of loss and degradation, she embodies grace.

Moss' 'Raft' is in my mind: the raft is the industry that keeps afloat the sick and their healers, with such grotesque results. As I attend to my patients here in Alice, I realise that I am one of those whose task is to help to steady the raft, to help keep it on course, to keep it straight on course to disaster.

2. CULTURED PEARLS

In 1991 I and a bunch of descendants of a family of pearling masters made our first visit to Broome. My ancestors were three brothers from Melbourne who set out together to find their fortune. Would they join a gold rush or go pearling? They tossed a coin: heads! – off to Broome for the pearls.

We went looking for records of the family's romantic past. We visited the museum, the courthouse, Chinatown, the Roebuck Hotel, all the old haunts. We found records of our old men everywhere. We rode out to Willie Creek to see and hear how they culture pearls in the modern-day pearling business of Broome.

We joined a couple of busloads of tourists sitting on the grass in the shade and listened to their host, an easy raconteur, as he described the seedy glamour of the past. Amusing, laconic, a lanky man beneath a suitably shabby hat, he held his audience in his palm. He regaled us with tales of past terrors, of tempest and shipwreck, of wartime bombings, of knifings in Chinatown, of death and agony from the bends, of casualties and victors in the quest for the pearl.

Now the speaker brings us to the present day. He gestures toward the nearby hiding place of a very large croc. 'Toothy', he calls him, casually domesticating the terrifying. He points out the spot in Willie Creek where illegal foreign fishers and trochus shell poachers are held. He recites the harm caused by these 'foreigners'. A murmur, a nodding of heads among his listeners.

Then to the science and technology of cultured pearling in the Broome of today. The speaker has a wonderful ability to render complicated material accessible. The audience learns of the scale, the value to Australia of the modern industry. They appreciate the dedication, the pioneer grit, the enterprise of ordinary Aussies who brought this industry back to life after the damage of World War II and the wreckage of the Depression. It is pleasant to contemplate the ripeness, the rightness of the present prosperity.

The speaker mentions a curious new phenomenon in the west – land rights claims in which Aboriginal groups lay claim to ancestral lands and 'sacred sites'. The speaker makes the quotation marks clearly audible. The audience smiles.

In the Kimberley, local groups are lodging claims too. Around Broome there is a claim for the coastline, both the seafront and the waters. The speaker smiles, makes a joke about possibly losing his farm, about the sudden proliferation of sacred sites, sites previously unheard of. But what would he know? He's lived here only sixty years …

The speaker pauses. His pleasant demeanour does not waver. He responds to questions from the audience:

Yeah, it is a bit sudden, all this indigenous spirituality.

And …

No madam, around here, there aren't many Aboriginal people who work. I wouldn't either, I guess. You know and I know – it's a lovely life up here. A drink or two, a lie down in the sun or in the shade, the fishing. Who'd work – so long as those welfare cheques keep coming in?

And …

Well, sir, they've got advisers and lawyers and government administrators. They get subsidies, they get grants, they get everything they ask for. It's a very powerful thing, very well resourced, this spirituality. Our small business would be outgunned in a land claim hearing. I'm considering changing the colour of my skin before the claim is heard.

More murmurs, knowing smiles, heads nodding all around.

No dissent.

The talk is finished. The speaker invites his guests to come inside the showroom, to have some refreshments and have a look at the pearls and local jewellery.

Everyone gets up, stretches, traipses off to the showroom. The host raconteur wanders off to a tap, connects up a hose and starts to water the shrubs that dot his pleasant lawns. One person from his audience materialises on the grass, approaches him, thanks and congratulates him on an entertaining talk, on his gift for anecdote and humour. Then he says, 'We lapped it up. We couldn't get enough of it. You really held us … That's why you were wrong to speak in that disrespectful way of my people and beliefs.'

'Me? Disrespectful? What are you talking about?'

'You have a gift. You speak and people listen. You joke and people laugh. People find you likeable. I do. Everyone who hears you wants to agree with you. Seventy, eighty people will leave here today, all feeling okay about ridiculing Aboriginal belief, all cynically convinced that it is money that is sacred, not land.'

'That's nonsense! Look, I've lived here all my life, I went to school with them, I've always lived close with Aborigines. I've got Aboriginal friends living over that dune there. We eat at each other's places every week. I'm not a racist.'

'Well, then, let me ask you a question: would you speak to your Aboriginal friends as you did to us? Would you make those jokes while they were your guests?'

'Ah … well … ah … no. Perhaps you are right. Perhaps I did go a bit far …'

The unpleasant visitor thanks his host and walks off. Not of Aboriginal descent, the visitor can in truth only refer to Aborigines as 'my people' from some sort of sentiment or belief. Perhaps the sentiment or belief is inherited.

After his pearling days were over, one of my ancestors stayed on in Broome and opened a law practice. Broome was a white supremacist town, unselfconscious and unashamed. Power was concentrated in the hands of the big pearlers. Few would oppose them.

My ancestor was safely white, but Jewish. He did not belong to the ruling clique. He was the only lawyer in town prepared to represent Japanese and Aboriginal clients in their cases against Europeans.

3. SHAKING HANDS WITH THE WRONG FOOT

I've been working in the Ngaanyatjarra Lands now for a couple of weeks, in the vastness of the Central Desert in Western Australia.

Each day I fly in to a new community and work closely with the local nurse. It would be truer to say I work under the direction of the nurse. She or he is everything of Medicine here for all but the six hours of the doctor's weekly visit. Trauma, infection, heart attack, intoxication, haemorrhage, epidemic chlamydia or syphilis, madness, cancer, birth and death – all are the province of the nurse. There are no off-duty days, there is no hour of any day or night when the nurse is not on call.

The doctor is useful for signing forms. I sign forms usefully, then we discuss problematic patients. The answers, the right decisions are invariably the nurse's suggestions.

During my short visit to the clinic, I see all the patients that the nurse – in this case, Stephen – has saved up for the doctor over the past week. As each patient comes in, Stephen makes a brief introduction: 'Hello, Robert, Howard is our doctor today.'

I say, 'Hello, Robert.' I am careful to look in his general direction but not to stare at him. I avoid direct eye contact.

I offer my hand, Robert gives me his. I clasp and shake. The patient's hand is passive, a passenger in my hand as it pumps an empty limb. When I speak, I try to do so clearly and slowly in shortish sentences. I avoid medical jargon. I choose concrete terms rather than abstractions. I do not rush him. I give him the time he needs.

We have our consultation in which the principal history-giver is the nurse. I prescribe or advise or treat, the patient gets up to go and once again we – rather I – shake hands.

After the morning session Stephen says, 'I see you shake hands with all the patients.'

'Yes.'

'Why?'

(Good question. It's what I do wherever I go, whomever I meet, barring strictly observant Jewish and Muslim women.)

'Well, I do it from habit, from instinct really. It starts with respect, with equality. It boils down to a physical offer and physical acceptance between two persons.'

'Yeah, maybe … but you notice the people here don't offer you their hand? Why do think that is?'

'They do give me their hand – once I've offered mine. I imagine they're simply shy or reserved.'

Maybe. The only time I've seen Ngaanyatjarra people shake hands with each other is at a sorry business.'

'You mean, after a death.'

'Yeah. Every person that you shake hands with here is reminded of death, of an evil spirit … and they're highly superstitious people to start with.'

'Good morning, nice to meet you. I'm Doctor Death.'

4. AFTER ULURU

'… There's been a death.'

I am in my small house in Yulara, cooking for *shabbat* on a Friday in December 2006, when the phone rings. A male voice speaks: 'It's Sergeant Benjamin, Doctor, of the Mutitjulu Police … I'm sorry to trouble you … there's been a death.'

A pause.

The voice resumes: 'It was a hanging. We need someone to certify the death. The nurses here can't do it; it has to be a doctor. I am sorry, Doctor.'

The voice is careful, it is feeling its way. I don't know the officer. The voice I hear is sober – sobered almost to a halt by the news of a death.

I ask the officer to bring the body to the clinic. We arrange to meet in twenty minutes' time.

It is early evening – 1830 hours in official language – when they pull up at the clinic. Even at that hour the heat is relentless. The sky is painted blue. There are two vehicles, a police car followed by an ambulance in its familiar livery of white slashed with red. A large oblong man steps out of a police car of such startling blueness that the sky pales behind it. The officer's face is deeply creased.

We shake hands.

His offsider gets out and straightens. She dwarfs her sergeant.

Apart from the odd post-adolescent pimple, her face is smooth. She walks over to the ambulance and commences a laughing conversation with the nurses who have driven the body.

After a time the nurses are free to attend to my questions. I address the older of the two, the one I know from the clinic: 'When was she found?'

She turns to her associate. For a moment, both are silent, then she says, 'I'm not really sure. The family called us an hour ago – when they felt ready to let us take the body, I guess. Someone found her before that and called the family. We don't know when …'

We release the latches and the heavy door of the ambulance clunks open, revealing a large white bag resting on a collapsed stretcher. Warm air flows from the interior.

The nurses step backward. Fumbling, I try to pull the stretcher a distance from the vehicle's dark interior. The nurses step forward and help, then again retreat. I pull on the zipper and the bag falls open, exposing the head and upper body of a human.

I pause. No sound, no movement.

There is a moment of reverent peacefulness. The skin of the person whom I stand and regard is brown, the same brown that glows from the earth and the many heads of rock in the early sunshine during my early morning run. That colour has penetrated me, claiming me like a mother.

I place the back of my gloved hand against the brown skin. It is still warm. Just as shocking, the face is very small.

I straighten and ask the nurses, 'Do you have a date of birth?'

One shows me a file. She points upper left, where I read, '19 November, 1991'.

I look again at the small face. There are a couple of blotches of acne. The child has buckteeth. The body is short and slender, the body of a girl who has scarcely begun the journey to womanhood.

I have no doubt, I feel no hope, but I rest my fingers lightly over her carotid artery. It is still.

I check her eyes. Dull now, pupils wide, fixed and unresponsive to the light – *those are pearls that were her eyes.*

I apply my stethoscope to her chest. The silence of death is drowned in a distracting chorus of inanimate rustling and chafing sounds. These are the artefacts of my examination. I hear no heartbeat. No air moves in or out of the chest.

This is the body of a fifteen-year old girl whose life is extinct.

No motion has she now, no force;

She neither hears nor sees;

Rolled round in earth's diurnal course,

With rocks, and stones, and trees.

I have another question for the nurses: 'What do you know of her health before today?'

'Six months back she was sniffing, but not since then; there's been no sniffable petrol in the community since then … There were some family problems. She had been seen by Mental Health …'

The answer is unsatisfactory. Any possible answer would be unsatisfactory. It all boils down to one thing: we do not know.

On an afterthought I lean forward again, peering past the fine cheekbones and the slender jaw, peering at the soft tissues beyond. There, on her throat I see what had to be seen, a bracelet patterned in her flesh, a curvilinear design that is unexpectedly graceful. It is the embossing in her skin of the fatal rope.

◎◎◎

After my time in Uluru, I return to practice in the city where life is conducted discreetly, where emergency services screen the ugly and the violent from us good citizens, and life feels normal again. Here the tragic is not the rule.

Half a year later, I am ready to work again in a remote community. I fly to Halls Creek in the Kimberley, dimly aware that the town is said to be 'troubled'.

As I board the plane, the hostie hands me a morning paper. Headlines leap out at me, reporting an alarming increase in youth suicide in the outback, especially in the Kimberley.

When I arrive in Halls Creek I am greeted by a passing parade of silent figures, most of them too thin or too fat, floating noiselessly like spirits along the streets of their own town, as if they have no right to be there. Or no right to be heard.

At night, it is the opposite: the people are heard, but darkskinned in the moonless dark, not readily seen. They cry out hoarsely, harshly, sounds of abuse, the odd scream, cries punctuated by peals of riotous laughter.

Late at night, sober people do not walk the streets in Halls Creek.

I go to work in the clinic. My patients seem to fall into two categories – those who are wrecked but salvageable and those who are wrecked, whom I cannot redeem. I work hard with members of the former group. Bare feet have been nicked by a bindi eye and have become infected. Scabies have been scratched and infection has entered. A small cut on a child's palm is infected.

At every infected site pus gathers. Where infection is deep set, the pus is trapped and it is my job to release the foul fluid. It pours, it bursts, stinking into freedom. The smell lingers in the air.

My patient feels relief and I, little relieved, bandage the foot, the hand, the leg, and send it out to become infected again.

And turn then to the unredeemed, to the old ones.

A ravaged woman, thin, hobbling on the arm of her stronger sister, her mind seemingly destroyed along with her body, is unable to recall how old her baby is. Her file tells me she is thirty-one years of age.

After two days at work in Halls Creek, I have contracted an insidious condition that is rampant in the town. Apathy and acceptance, braided into a noose, rest around the neck here. Slowly, it tightens into a passivity that numbs and deadens. I have never before been afflicted in this way.

You can get the papers here, one day late. Page after page is full of gloomy reports of the Aboriginal condition, page after page of relentless criticism of the industry in which I work as a reliever for a palliator.

And although Halls Creek is a town of only 1800 souls, the name appears with surprising frequency on the pages of this Perth daily. Halls Creek appears to be proverbial for all the things that have gone wrong, everything that has been done, everything that has been done wrongly, everything that has not been done.

The paper arrives twenty-four hours late, but it makes no difference. Not until Thursday 21 June 2007. That is the day when the Prime Minister shakes off his own passivity and declares martial law against child abuse in the Northern Territory.

I feel confused. I am not surprised to find myself deeply ambivalent about these brave, bold, brash initiatives. For anyone with any humility, confusion is morally mandatory in Aboriginal matters. And confusion is, of course, quite useless.

But no one else I speak to seems confused. Among people who are not customarily supporters of the Prime Minister, minds are quickly made up: it has to be done.

Today is Friday. There are new regulations in Halls Creek that restrict the sale of grog. You can't buy alcohol before midday and you aren't allowed to buy more than a dozen cans of full-strength beer. A few minutes after noon I pass the bottle shop as a stream of people snakes along the road. The new grog regulations are taking effect – everyone carries the identical purchase; everyone has bought the maximum.

Early this evening there will be a footy match in town. There is a mob coming from near the Northern Territory border to play the local team. (I try to imagine Collingwood going to play in

Sydney – the whole team driving both ways. Next weekend, the home teams will drive similar distances for their away matches.) Here is an opportunity to see something distinctive, an exhibition of gifts in full and exuberant flower. Aboriginals playing footy are not known for passivity.

I decide to walk the 150 metres to the town's floodlit oval. An emerald of green, it shines in the light, a reminder of how grass used to look in the country towns of the Garden State.

Although it is only 6.00 p.m. the town is dark and drunk and very easily audible. At the corner of Hall Street and the Northern Highway, a man urinates against a fence. At the next corner a woman stands beneath a street light, her shirt undone, her breasts fully exposed to view. She stands there, more or less steadily, her back braced against the fence, facing the street. Is she offering herself for sale? Or is she available free of charge? Or is she simply too drunk to achieve the buttoning of a shirt, or just unconscious of her exposure?

The night is rent with the cries of kids, the screams of women, the hoonish menace of daylight's shy youths as they bay now in groups to an unseen moon.

I never make it to the footy. After a few minutes I turn and retreat to my house, to the peace and sweetness of *shabbat*.

5. LAND OF THE MAGPIE GEESE

The last night of my first locum. Tomorrow the regular doctor will return to his practice and I'll drive from Kakadu to Darwin then fly back south. At midnight the phone rings. The voice on the phone is talking about a man with a cut head. 'He dived into a pool …'

The soft clouds of sleep part and I begin to remember that I am a doctor, *the* doctor. A head injury following a dive … has he injured his spine?

Minutes later I meet the man with the 'cut head' at the clinic. Beginning above one ear, the laceration traverses his skull to the back of the opposite eyebrow. He has been half scalped. There is surprisingly little bleeding; the skull, exposed, dull white, is a confession.

The man makes light of his injury. 'Just bung in a coupla stitches, Doc. Nothing serious. I wasn't gunna come … musta been a bit stunned … me mate here bunged me into the four wheel. Wouldna bothered, meself …'

The man isn't a local. He has been shooting a feature movie up here, filmed all day, returned, hot and tired and thirsty to the pub, had a few drinks, ate dinner, had a few more drinks, then, 'Felt like a swim, dived in, banged me head … shallower than I thought. Just stitch me up, Doc, I'll get outa ya hair.'

The man is in his late thirties. Good-looking, fair, well made, he smells of alcohol and Dutch courage. The movie man is acting a part. Tonight he is the laconic frontiersman.

I spend a good while checking body parts remote from his cut head. Sensation, power, reflexes in both upper limbs – all are assessed. All intact. The man's brain works too. But I'm uneasy. That scalped head took a mighty belt. The cut skin edges aren't bleeding because the impact squashed the blood vessels closed. Who knows whether his spine has been injured?

When I palpate the back of the man's neck, he is irritable. 'Doc, it's me head that's hurt, not me neck or me bloody hands. Just stitch me up and let me go.'

Ignorant, insubordinate, stubborn, I persist, probing for telltale tenderness in the vertebrae of the neck. The man watches me minutely. He sees a man who refuses to play along, a man worrying about something big.

No longer laconic, now nakedly hostile, this is a man whose anxiety has become stronger than the grog.

The angry man and the difficult doctor spend the next five hours in each other's company. The doctor and the nurse are preparing for the man's retrieval by the Royal Flying Doctor Service. The man protests when I forbid him to bend or move his neck; he growls as we apply the collar; and he complains loudly into his mobile phone about 'the bloody doctor, an old bloody woman, he's shipping me out to Darwin – that prick wouldn't have a clue what this delay will mean to the movie – and he still won't stitch up my bloody cut.'

But eventually the man, sobering, complies. He protects his neck, he accepts referral to the surgeon for the cut head. Meanwhile the nurse and the doctor watch and monitor the man's vital signs closely.

Around 3 a.m. a small lady comes into the clinic, clutching a dishcloth to a cut head. She has few words.

Beneath a good light the lady looks about sixty. Her face is wrinkled and scarred. This morning's injury is a jagged, deepish cut that snakes down her forehead, between her eyes to the bridge of her nose. Her nose is swollen, perhaps broken.Her name – the name she gives us – is Sylvia.

This lady is a guest of the Crocodile Hotel, just across the lawns from the clinic. She had taken a room in the hotel, but she'd decided not to sleep there; it was too cold in the airconditioning. So she and her man came outside and slept on the grass.

She woke, disturbed by someone rifling her pockets and groping for her purse. This lady receives royalty money. She is a traditional owner of land where they are mining uranium.

She fended off the thief, a man – her man. He had been drinking in the hotel. He was full but he wanted more grog.

He humbugged her. She refused. He persisted, found her implacable, looked for something to make her see reason. He sighted a suitable implement on the edge of the grass. It was a star picket …

We clean the wound, gently inject the local anaesthetic, carefully trim away dead skin, fish out bits of the Crocodile Hotel garden, appose the skin edges and attempt to restore her face. She lies still while I insert a score of fine sutures, and makes no complaint. Sylvia is impassive as we ask whether she wants to lay charges. She is indifferent to our referral to the Domestic Violence worker. I write a detailed report of her injuries in case she decides to see the police. It takes me longer to write a legible report than it took to repair her wounds.

She crushes the report into a pocket and goes outside, back to her man.

The Flying Doctor arrives at the airport and the ambos drive the movie man away. A suspected fractured neck and partial scalping are not everyday diagnoses in general practice. A facial laceration is mundane. But it is Sylvia with her cut face who weighs the more heavily as I drive to Darwin and then fly south. And eighteen years on, it is Sylvia who weighs upon me still.

6. BY THE RIVERS OF EDEN

Now a river went out of Eden
To water the garden …

(Genesis 2:10)

I travel north from Melbourne's grey winter to Katherine, where it is hot and humid, and there are blue skies. There is a river here, also named Katherine. I stroll along the river bank and quickly I am back in my childhood home in the Riverina. I look up and there, caught in the topmost branches of high eucalypts, I sight a camp chair, plastic bags and a riot of planks. This flotsam from the last summer's floods is ten metres above today's river level.

Those floods were colossal. Katherine was a brown sea, the hospital an island, the town a daily TV spectacle before an amazed nation. Here was an Australian town, underwater, like something you see in the Third World.

☺☺☺

I begin working in the hospital's Casualty Department. My first patient is a woman in late middle age who has a kidney infection. She lies still and stoical through the prolonged admission procedures, her pain still untreated.

I discover with shock that her actual age is thirty-eight years. She has left her six children in the care of her sister in a remote

Aboriginal community, some hundreds of kilometres distant from here. In addition to her infection, she has diabetes and advanced heart disease, the latter due to damage to a heart valve resulting from rheumatic fever. Rheumatic heart disease is uncommon in my work in the city, but here it is commonplace, a consequence of ordinary everyday scabies infected by ordinary everyday strep. I learn that scabies is constant, a gift from ubiquitous dogs, intimately present, day and night.

Her medical file is thick with admissions such as this, the most recent only three weeks ago. On that occasion, too, illness took her from her children.

As I work through this lady's diseases, raised voices and hoarse swearing break into the room. The police escort a man, noisily drunk, whose forehead and temple have born jaggedly torn open by a nulla nulla.

'Were you knocked out?' I need to know.

The man looks at me. He does not speak.

I try again. The man looks in my general direction, but our eyes and our minds do not meet.

Both the club and alcohol have given his brain a fearful thumping. He is unable to give me any history. I do not speak his language.

I clean and stitch up the surface wounds, worrying and wondering whether there are internal wounds inside his skull that I have not detected. Is there a small blood vessel, broken and leaking, with blood gathering to a brain-crushing mass that will kill or cripple him?

Well before I finish, my patient is snoring. He remains in a stupor for most of the day. After he awakens the police will take him away to a shelter to sober up.

A phone call from the local Aboriginal Health Centre warns of the imminent arrival of a man who fell asleep and rolled into a fire and stayed asleep.

When they bring him into the hospital, he is barely awake. We roll up the charred fabric of his trousers, exposing a white 'sock' of pallid, bloodless muscle tissue that has been cooked. The flesh falls away in large lumps, exposing naked bone – an obscene sight. The patient is impassive, the nurses intent. Among those present, only this city doctor appears shocked.

At the end of my day's shift I go for a run – from the hospital into town – a distance of four kilometres. I run past the roadside sign offering treatment for drug and alcohol problems; I run past the School of the Air, which bills itself as 'the world's largest class-room'; I run until I reach Red Rooster and pull up suddenly to avoid the unconscious figures of two adults, dead drunk, their bodies intertwined, lying on the footpath in front of me.

We are here in the middle of the town. No one can miss the sight I see, but no one pays heed.

I visit the post office and stand in the queue. I look up as a sudden scuffing and scrambling sound from the head of the line disturbs the peace. There is a man engaged in a slow motion wres-tling match with a stack of cartons and a cardboard display. The cartons fall and the man bounces from one to another to the floor, tries to rise, falls again, and lies back. He looks up at us shoppers and flashes a big smile, then declares, with a sort of comic candour: 'TOO DRUNK!'

☺☺☺

Back at the hospital, I check on my patient with the head injury. He is still asleep. His vital signs are fine: there is no sign of an internal haemorrhage.

I sit for a while and muse on pervasive lack of self-care. I fret about a language that I do not have. I look up at the clock on the wall. The thought occurs to me: does this man who sleeps inhabit the same time as mine? Does my time – with its before and after – create distinct understandings? Of cause and effect, and of prevention?

Is this man indifferent to my time?

Deep in mocking sleep, oblivious of all perplexity and regret, and of all subtle cultural speculation, my patient enjoys his rest.

7. UN DIDGE AUTENTICO

My relative, Damian, manufactures and sells exotic musical instruments, including didgeridoos, in Capilla del Monte, a small town on a hilltop in Cordoba in Argentina. He says he wants 'a real didgeridoo, Howardo. One that expresses the maker's soul. *Un didge autentico*'.

This might not be straightforward: sometimes a didge is not a didge; sometimes it's a *yidaki*. And sometimes it's made of the wrong material, or by the wrong people, or by the wrong method, or …

I ask Albert at the hospital for guidance. Albert is a local, a Jawoyn, certainly authentic himself. He is a trained health worker who also doubles as mortuary attendant here – a busy portfolio.

Albert's advice: 'Go to the main streets and look around at the didgeridoos in the shops. Then come and tell me what you see and what you like. Don't buy anything!'

I do as Albert advises and I find a shop filled with attractive objects and art works. They are labelled; most are local, but the most inexpensive come from Newcastle. None of them comes from China.

I like them, I like the prices, I even like the hard old nut with the authentic blue rinse who is the brisk saleslady. Her sales pitch is direct: 'If you like it, buy it; otherwise don't waste my time.'

I do like, I don't buy. I return to Albert and report.

'Good thinking, Doc. A Newcastle didgeridoo is as authentic as blue hair: no indigenous people ever made didgeridoos south of Alice. And no woman ever played a didge in ceremony; a woman doesn't have that law.'

Albert sketches a mud map for me. 'Go to this place. It's out of town a bit, closer to us here at the hospital.'

The out-of-town-a-bit place is close – compared to Alice or Newcastle. By the time I arrive on foot I am pretty hot and dry. The place looks like someone's garage, which it is. I ask the old codger sitting in the shade where the didge shop is. He points his thumb backwards over his left shoulder. I go inside, envying him his can of fruit juice.

Inside there are lots of pictures for sale, but no didges. A bloke appears and offers advice. He is immediately sympathetic to my quest for not just any old didge but an authentic one. 'You've come to the right place, mate. All our didges are dinkum, all local, all made from the right wood, harvested right, made by the right people.'

His words are encouraging but his marked New Zealand accent is a worry. Guardedly, I ask, 'What would be wrong wood?'

'Has to be eucalypt, should be eaten out by termites then hollowed with hot coal. No bamboo.'

'Why no bamboo? I've read that bamboo was the original wood …'

'Not for a didge, mate; that's a *yidaki*. The Yolngu make them, up in Arnhem Land. Down here and everywhere south of here, they're didgeridoos. But no didgeridoo can be older than a hundred years.'

I know that can't be correct. The didgeridoo is the oldest continuously played instrument in the world. I share this datum with Mister Kiwi.

He nods and grins then shakes his head. 'Quite right, mate. But they only started *calling* them didgeridoos a hundred years back.

The didge is the generic name. It's new. In Kakadu it's a *garnbak*; in the Kimberley it's a *ngaribi*; the Arrente call it *ilpirra*; in the Cobourg Peninsula it's called *wuyimba*: that's the word for trachea. And so on ... Here the Jawoyn mob call it *artawirr*, which means hollow log. Anyway, I'm not the right person to tell you or show you this.'

'You're not? You're pretty knowledgeable for a man from somewhere else.'

'Yeah, mate, but my sort of knowledge isn't understanding. And anyway, some knowledge is secret. You want an initiated man ... There is an old man in this community, very senior in the Law, who makes didges for ceremony. He doesn't make many. He decorates them too, nothing fancy or intricate. Simple, not pretentious.' He smiles. 'That's your authentic man. He's not a talker. He's not commercial, he's a Law man. He's not your everyday person.'

'Where will I find him? As a matter of interest, where will I find your didges? I don't see any.'

The knowledgeable man smiles and leads me outside. He introduces me to the elderly man in the shade. They speak, then the old man gets up and walks slowly to a shed, opens it, sits down on the earthen floor and bent-thumb points to the dozen or so didgeridoos behind him. He sucks on his fruit juice in silence.

I look at the didges, all of them heavy, non-bamboo articles, their motifs pleasant enough, if a bit plain.

I ask him, 'What does that design mean?'

'Rainbow serpent, here she sleeping underground. 'Ere. She wake up, she push up, up, come out of ground, up on top ... travel, travel, she get tired, rest. 'Ere ...'

The old man's speech is indistinct, a bit disjointed. I am unsure whether or not I follow him.

Whenever he says 'ere the old man prods a stumpy finger at his design. Now he falls silent, takes another drink and remains silent.

I'd like to know more, but I'm not certain of the etiquette. Is this material secret? Diffidently I ask, 'Can you tell me anything more?'

'All that meaning here … 'E say 'ere sleeping, 'ere travelling. Leave tracks. Come back … 'Ere tickle frogs, tickle stomach. Frogs laugh …' – and the old man laughs, a wheezy laugh that becomes a cough, then a coughing fit, then a hefty spit. He resumes, 'Water come out … track 'ere make river, tracks 'ere, and 'ere, make lakes.'

The old man's speech is a mumble. All his talk of water makes him dry. He drinks again. I'm a bit dry too. I look more closely at his orange juice can. I read Vodka and Orange.

In the silence, I begin to wonder: is this authentic lore, law in fact? Or is it all authentic drunken rambling? Is this old man just another purveyor of grog art?

''E say 'ere, water wake up fish, wake up animal, big one, little one, mother, granny, grandpa, grass, bird, tree … All that big animal, all that little one …'

I can hardly hear him, and I certainly don't understand.

And that's all I will learn today.

I do buy a didge for Damian. Who can know whether it's ridgy-didge or a dodgy didge?

☉☉☉

Postscript: I Google 'Dreaming in Katherine'. At www.culture.gov.au, I follow some prompts and read the following:

> The Jawoyn people, of the Katherine Gorge area in the Northern Territory, tell how the Rainbow Serpent slept under the ground until she awoke in the Dreaming and pushed her way to the surface. She travelled the land, sleeping when she tired, and left behind her winding tracks and the imprint of her sleeping body. When she had travelled the earth she returned and called to the frogs to come out, but they were very slow because their bodies were full of water. The rainbow serpent tickled their stomachs and when the frogs laughed the

water flowed out of their mouths and filled the tracks and hollows left by the Rainbow Serpent, creating the rivers and lakes. This woke all the animals and plants, who then followed the Rainbow Serpent across the land.

PART TWO

NEXT DOOR TO
PARADISE

Four sages entered paradise.
One cast a glance and died; one looked and went mad;
another mutilated the shoots. Only Rabbi Akiva
entered in peace and departed in peace.

(Extracted and paraphrased from Tractate Chagiga, P14b)

8. THE VALLEY OF THE PROPHETS

Balgo is a desert community in Western Australia that sits on the edge of a secret. Hidden here from the eyes of an incurious world is a grand topographic feature, the Pound – a vast dished area with raised edges. Its huge red walls of crag and tumbled rock are a reminder of the insignificance of a mortal being; in all this grandeur a human is an insect.

From a secular geological perspective the Pound is simply a depression, a mere shovel mark on the earth's surface. But the locals are far from secular. An ancient people living in a wilderness of blasting heat and red rock, they have long held the Catholic Church in affection. And the people have a particular attachment to biblical names.

At the geometric centre of this very small town is the footy oval, a sort of sacred site. Every building in town genuflects towards the footy ground. Only the Catholic Church, a stone building, towers high above it. Outside the church is a statue of Jesus in white stone, clad in a mantle of scarlet. He stands opposite the full forward position, his arms held out and open before him in an attitude of either compassion or of readiness to accept a pass into the forward line. The clinic where I work is situated on the wing.

In the course of my first morning at the clinic, I meet Elijah and Micah and Isaiah and Zachariah. In a roll call of Old Testament prophets, I also meet and treat Moses, Hezekiah and Nathan. And

Nicodemus, whom I do not recognise from that canon.

Elijah is a splendid-looking youth. Aged nineteen, he is lean and muscular. With his full lips and fine teeth, his face is built for smiling. But he is not smiling now. In fact, he can barely speak or move his facial muscles. He cradles an ice pack against his right temple and cool towels swathe his forehead and cheek. I remove these coverings and find blistered skin and raw patches where the skin falls away in sheets.

These are fresh burns.

Moving is difficult for Elijah, because his ribs and abdomen are sore. Speaking is hard because of his burns. His aunt, who has sat impassively by him, now speaks: 'He copped a kicking. They kicked him all over. Then they threw a kettle of boiling water over him.'

I look at Elijah's face. A broad band of scald extends from the right side of his scalp, down the forehead and face, onto the chin and neck. The ear has been cooked. Somehow, by some reflex, his right eyelids sheltered Elijah's eye and saved it.

Why, I wonder, did they do all this?

The police interview Elijah as we dress his burns. He complains of cough. I listen to his chest and hear rattling sounds. He has a fever too. But despite his pounded and parboiled state, he looks surprisingly well – too well perhaps for this to be pneumonia, but I treat him for that contingency – just in case.

The next day, the blistering is worse. On the morning of the third day, dead skin is lifting, exposing pink skin underneath. Elijah is starting to look like Michael Jackson. But he looks well and he can speak now without pain.

◎◎◎

A nurse asks me to see Zachariah. He came in with a spot of pus on his left elbow. When she started to mop up the bead of pus with some moistened gauze, the skin fell away. The tissues underneath were dead too. The more the nurse cleaned, the deeper and wider became the exposed area, until the bones of the elbow were exposed, horrifyingly. Like me, the nurse is a newcomer to the clinic. She is alarmed by what she sees.

As I inspect the elbow, I feel like a witness to obscenity.

I read Zachariah's clinical notes. This elbow has been cleansed, disinfected and smothered in antibiotics and dressed, every few weeks for *five years*! And the elbow has not healed.

One of the veteran nurses fills in the gaps: 'We clean the elbow and treat it. He agrees to come back the next day for re-dressing, but then we don't see Zachariah for a fortnight. He goes on a bender, falls asleep on the earth, his elbow mouldering underneath him. It happens again and again. He can't help himself. And we can't cure him.'

◎◎◎

Noah has a face that looks ready to explode into laughter. I pick him for about seventy, but he's forty-four. He shambles across the gravel oval to the clinic, listing to starboard, his right arm tucked in next to his body like a close-hauled sail. His face is skew-whiff, distorted into spurious joviality by the head injury he suffered five years ago in a single-vehicle road accident. Unassuming, gentle, he sits with imperturbable patience and waits his turn to be seen.

Recently, the tip of his right third finger was amputated. A surgeon trimmed and dressed the stump; now Noah comes to have the dressing changed. Aged and discoloured, the present dressing looks an ancient artefact, a museum piece. We remove it gently and find a lake of pus beneath the skin, extending backwards the entire length of what remains of the finger. That digit is doomed, the hand itself is now under threat.

Noah was due to see us twelve days ago but, like his Biblical namesake, he was waylaid by the drink and fell asleep.

◉◉◉

The CEO of Balgo Health takes me to one side. 'There's a bloke here we need you to see. He's senior in the Law here, beautiful fella, his wife's the same. He's dying of liver disease … it's tragic. He's not old, but he's the senior man – in this country.

'He doesn't often come in to the clinic and when he does, we don't like to keep him waiting. Everyone here – his own people and all of us at the clinic – everyone loves him, everyone looks up to him. Never hurt anyone in his life, only himself, with the grog.'

The CEO takes me to a private room and introduces me to Moses and Deborah. Moses gives me a cool dry hand. The fingernail beds are blue. His full beard is grey, his face too; only his eyes are yellow. He breathes rapidly through pale lips and his breath is shortened by his vast abdominal girth. This is not fat but ascitic fluid, gathering inside his abdominal cavity from an endless seeping. His body fluids are 'thinned' for lack of the serum proteins that his failing liver can no longer create.

I look at him and try an encouraging smile, a wordless lie. His wife catches my look. Her eyes widen with hope. But Moses looks back at me squarely and truly. He knows.

He needs only a repeat of his fluid tablets. Those are not holding back the waters. He asks for nothing more, expects nothing. He holds my hand and he thanks me with simple dignity, as if I had made a difference. He is simply being kind, kind to the living.

I feel a heavy sadness.

◉◉◉

One after another, the casualties of grog come in to see us.

This takes me by surprise. The first thing I saw on landing at the Balgo airstrip was the notice declaring Balgo a dry community. The language on the notice is culturally assertive. A visitor reads and understands that the locals make the rules here. A permit is required merely to visit. This looks like a community whose leaders have taken their salvation into their own hands.

But so many of these patients are damaged by alcohol.

Then the policeman explains, 'We had the Balgo sports carnival this weekend. All the communities as far east as Yuendumu came here. The place was flooded with alcohol.'

There is another puzzle – the apparent cyclic regularity of grog casualties seen at the clinic; they seem to come in fortnightly. Does this correspond to the arrival of welfare cheques? The policeman nods and adds, 'The grog runners time their visits for pension day ... so do the drug smugglers.'

◎◎◎

On the third night, Elijah turns up at the clinic in an animated state. He has some news for me and for the rest of the clinic: 'I am Satan's boss. I cannot die. I have special powers. I can see the future.'

This is a new Elijah. He wears a t-shirt of brilliant hues, all blazes of scarlet, jagged angles of black and streaks of gold. His rich head of black hair is confined by a bandana in red and gold. He is a lair in primary colours, an Aboriginal flag incarnate.

He tells the nurse, 'I know whatever you are thinking. I know everything that the doctor is thinking too.

'I drove my motor bike flat out and crashed into a house and got up and walked away. Nothing can hurt me.'

I ask Elijah, 'What about your bike? Was it damaged?'

'Doesn't matter. I have three motor bikes and two cars.'

Elijah paces about the Emergency Room as he speaks. He won't sit down. He has more to tell us: 'I can jump from the top of the Pound. I cannot die.'

The policeman whispers a chilling aside: 'He was at the Pound, pacing up and down at the edge, about to jump ... His cousin was there and grabbed him. His mother died a little while back.'

Hearing the word *mother*, Elijah turns to us and says, 'My mother is in heaven. I am the boss of Satan. Dogs run away from me because I am the devil. When I am drunk, I am sober, and when I am sober, I am drunk. Nothing can hurt me. I can't die.'

Elijah's burned face lights and beams as he speaks. Clearly, he is happy to tell us all this.

When I ask him to confirm this or that detail, he makes a clicking sound with his mouth. He is cocky, he shines assurance of his mastery of all he sees, and much that we cannot. In all Elijah's comic bravado I see the domestic tragedy of a boy who has lost his Mum and now has lost his mind.

The policeman has an additional insight: 'Elijah, were you on the grog this weekend?'

Elijah clicks a cheerful *'yes'*.

'What about ganja, Elijah?'

Another click, then he adds, 'I've had a couple of cones today.'

Ah yes, ganja – aka cannabis – that *soft* drug, the substance implicated in every single new psychotic illness that I have seen in the last twenty years.

I consult the *Manual of Psychiatric Emergencies* and offer Elijah some antipsychotic medication. He takes it cheerfully. Then he resumes pacing and talking at a hundred miles per hour. He is delightful and quite mad. Now I have a sense of the motivation of Elijah's assailants: perhaps he simply drove his friends crazy with his raving.

Eventually, Elijah subsides and allows himself to be taken away by an aunty who promises to bring him back to us in the morning. But I expect to see him as soon as the medication wears off. It could be a busy night.

Before I can commit a patient for involuntary treatment in Western Australia, there are three criteria which must be satisfied.

1. He must be psychotic. Elijah is that.
2. He must be a risk to others or to himself. Elijah – whom

nothing can harm, who was about to leap from the Pound – is certainly at risk.

3. He must refuse treatment. Here Elijah breaks the mould. He will do anything we ask. Most jocund apt and willing is he ...

I do not wish to commit Elijah to a psychiatric hospital. Always a violation of human dignity, committal here would be particularly unpleasant. The nearest psychiatric hospital is in Perth, a world away from the East Kimberley. Transfer must be by the Royal Flying Doctor Service. You can't have a madman running amok in a small aircraft, so the patient must be very heavily sedated and physically restrained. The restraints are a mesh of stout straps that immobilise the limbs at the ankles, knees, wrists and arms. There are numerous additional straps that bind the torso to a bed or stretcher in every direction, so that the patient is literally unable to have an erection.

With the patient now so comprehensively restrained and sedated, he must have a catheter inserted into his bladder for the hours of restraint. No one, mad or sane, enjoys the insertion of a urinary catheter. Finally, our patient will be too sleepy to eat or drink and, in addition, he might require immediate sedation, so an intravenous drip must be inserted into a vein. For safety's sake, the RFDS requires a drip in either arm.

I consider Elijah. He hasn't intimated, by word or action, any aggressive intent. He is the most harmless of patients. And the most vulnerable. At present I am treating him in Balgo (pop. 200), but he normally resides at Ringer's Soak (pop. eighty souls). If we knock him out, tie him up and fly him out to the city, he'll wake up in a place foreign to him beyond understanding. Is this necessary?

Here in Balgo, Elijah is attended by solicitous aunts and by his great-uncle and great-aunt, venerable people who show endless concern for him. This pacing Elijah, this prophesying Elijah is not the boy they know. He unsettles them. Instinctively, they wish to take him to Ringer's Soak, to see him safe back home. There, more aunties will care for him. Great-uncle says he'll drive Elijah today. I look at great-uncle. Great seems the right word for him: his face is surrounded by a crescent of silver beard, a halo inverted onto the lower half of his golden face; great, too, in girth. Great also in deeds – he with his wife is custodian of so many of their orphaned, damaged or detached descendants. Theirs is a life of endless, exhausting solicitude.

Ringer's Soak (the locals place the emphasis on the first word, where we English speakers would accentuate the second) is a metaphoric asylum only, a coming home of profound meaning but greater uncertainty. Ringer's Soak has one nurse, no doctor, no police. Over the phone the nurse is shrill in her urging: 'Fly him out, fly him out to where he'll be safe.'

There is a spare seat on tomorrow afternoon's flight to Halls Creek – my flight. Once I fly out on that plane Balgo will be left undoctored and facing a medico-legal problem. There will be no one here to certify a person insane and to order his committal.

An idea gleams: perhaps Elijah can be our fourth passenger tomorrow; I could take the medico-legal problem with me and win him a reprieve at Halls Creek Hospital. I am ready to warrant his docility. I get onto the phone and place a lot of long-distance, long-duration calls.

Before I even put this idea to my fellow passengers (who include a burly colleague), before I put it to my employers and to the CEO of Balgo Health, before I discuss it with the Kimberley regional psychiatrist, I can guess what they will say. And when the veto does come, it is unanimous and I bow to it. Why, I wonder, are doctors so timorous?

The police officers here are not timid. Big strong boys, experienced, good-humoured, they are genuinely respectful in a way that has nothing to do with political rectitude. Over the last twelve hours they have been murmuring muted offers to drive Elijah to Halls Creek. The drive is a mere 250 kilometres along the great

Tanami Track, that emblem of extremity in the Australian consciousness of country.

These blokes are not short of things to do back here in Balgo; like me, they want to help Elijah and to relieve his family.

The cops are willing, but it turns out that regulations forbid them to take a passenger in their car who is not either under arrest or certified insane. They have no insurance against a (highly likely) legal claim should anything go awry.

A day passes. Another day in which Elijah hears the voice telling him he has Satanic powers, another night and day in which he floats high then dreams deeply under my medication, while his anxious relatives watch over him; another day, another blazing t-shirt.

On the fourth evening, Elijah stops pacing. His speech slows briefly to a standstill. He looks squarely at me and speaks quietly. 'You've been good to me, Doc. I owe you one, bro.'

I look hard back at him, wondering whether this is the drug-prophet speaking, or whether this is some fugitive Elijah, fearing harm, sensing a protector. I fancy it is the former, but I do not know, and I will never know. The distinction matters, but only to me.

On the final morning, Elijah fails to make our 9 o'clock rendez-vous at the clinic. By 10.15 he has not appeared and there is no word. The nurse drives out to the camp of the aunties and brings him in. Another t-shirt, this the brightest of all, a technicolour dream with silver spangles across the breast. Elijah is a cool, cool dude. He tells me that my hat is cool, lifts my yarmulka from my head and puts it on his own. Elijah, his face all dappled with scald and peel and natural ebony, his smile transfiguring all – Elijah looks good in a yarmulka.

But he is still Satan's boss, still indestructible, still very much at risk.

Another idea rises uncertainly like a winter sun in the east of my mind. Perhaps *I* could drive Elijah along the Tanami Track to hospital in Halls Creek. I have reason to believe we all will be received in Halls Creek.

More telephony.

Yep, the over-worked, ever-helpful hospital doctor in Halls Creek will go along with it. Diffidently he requests that I will continue Elijah's care, once he is admitted. Easy.

The CEO at Balgo will release one of his few vehicles, a Toyota troop carrier, for the trip. He says yes, but he wonders how and when he'll get his troopie back.

Now I have a vehicle, a patient, and some doubts. What if Elijah needs my medical attention while I'm driving? What if we stop for a leak and Elijah absconds? I'll need to recruit additional muscle and experience.

A phone call to the local police chief, Anthony. I ask somewhat hesitantly, 'How would you feel about lending me an officer to come along for the ride – in an unofficial capacity – to ride shotgun with me?' I explain that I have completed the forms for Elijah's certification and committal in every particular save one: I have not signed them. Should the situation warrant it, I would sign and then the police officer could apply handcuffs and act, fully insured, in an official capacity.

Instantly he says yes. And he volunteers to do the job himself.

We arrange to leave at 2.00 p.m. They say the drive will take three and a half hours, so with luck we'll arrive before dusk, before every native animal comes out onto the roads to play chicken with our oncoming vehicle. The nurse, Brenda, will go and find Elijah at 1.00 p.m. and sedate him. Brenda has another good idea: she'll find a relative to travel with Elijah, indispensable for his peace of mind on leaving country.

◎◎◎

There is one thing I want to do before I leave this place. Balgo is famous Australia-wide for its Waylayirti Arts, the cooperative enterprise of local painters. At the end of the morning clinic, I duck out and visit their large premises, a high airy building, a sort of warehouse whose floors and walls are covered with large canvases. One work, hanging on the wall opposite the front door, takes my eye as I enter. It is about three feet by four and it consists of small painted dots. The dots swim in wide flowing currents from side to side and from bottom to top of the canvas. The blues flow into the greens, the yellows into the reds and pinks. The whole has a quiet, swelling, irresistible beauty.

It is love at first sight.

I have fallen in love in this way before and it has been awkward for me back home, later, as I have tried to explain to my wife.

I control myself.

I enquire about the price; that should cool me down. It doesn't – the painting is affordable.

The manager of the gallery explains that the painting is of bush tucker at Mulan, the settlement about thirty kilometres distant where I worked a couple of days ago. The dots represent a grain-bearing grass that grows around the lake at Mulan; the various colours depict the grain at different stages of ripening through the cycle of seasons. Local people grind and pound the grains into a flour which they bake into damper. The work is a homage to the manna of this area, the traditional staple.

I have not yet managed to cool down. I decide to look at some other works. There are hundreds and hundreds standing in vertical stacks and lying in heaps, and scores of larger works hanging on the walls. I scarcely find any that are not attractive and accomplished. If that first painting is love, then this place is a harem.

In a large room to one side of the gallery, a painter sits on the floor, surrounded by a riot of tubes of paint and brushes. Before him and to one side is a rectangle of plywood which serves as his palette. He bends forward and works on a large canvas which he is slowly covering with a tightly patterned series of geometric lines and curves. Using only a handful of pigments, broadly ochreous, he is creating something quite arresting. His first name is arresting too. It is Helicopter.

Sitting on a stool just by the door is a petite lady, very old, resting her thin back against a counter. Standing on the floor next to the stool is her four-point walking stick. I spend some time standing at the counter, arranging with the manager to send an email image of 'my' painting to my wife.

While I wait, I leaf through a catalogue of the gallery's entries in next week's Indigenous Art awards, to be held in Darwin. There I see a painting by one of the most famous names in Australian art. Next to it is a small photo of the artist and her CV. I read of her one-woman shows in Australia and abroad, and of her audience with the Queen. The face in the photo is the face of the small lady seated on my right. Here in Balgo I have stumbled across an international luminary, a hidden Malouf.

I race back to pack, my mind racing too, with the painters and paintings, with this trove of beauty amongst the ugliness, and with the new love in my life.

◎◎◎

At 2.00 p.m. we are all ready, all assembled at the clinic: Anthony, Brenda, cousin Ezekiel, the troopie, and me. But no Elijah. Brenda hasn't found him; that means he will remain unsedated for the drive along the Tanami.

No one is surprised, no one else seems dismayed.

Brenda introduces me to Ezekiel. Ezekiel is Elijah's age, a community warden, one who has accepted responsibilities, his brothers' keeper. He will travel on from Halls Creek 'for training'.

'Footy?' I ask.

'No, computers.'

I have a quiet word with Anthony, tell him of the injectable medications I have drawn up in syringes, ready for contingencies.

Says Anthony, 'I have pepper spray. If I have to use it, best you get out and away from the vehicle quickish.'

Ezekiel finds Elijah swiftly. Elijah swallows his tablets, climbs aboard and commences an animated one-sided conversation that will continue for seventy-five unnerving minutes.

A farewell drive to the Pound, that edge of the beyond, where Elijah heard the still soft voice. A final look out from the heights, now with the sun at its height, a straining into the glare. On my first drive out here I had not recognised this: it is the valley of the prophets.

A prompt U-turn, then we are off to the Tanami Track. The time is 2.30 p.m. Ezekiel sits next to me in the front. Elijah is immediately behind me, seated in my blind spot, separated from me by strong steel mesh. And Anthony's stout form occupies the space between Elijah and the back door.

For the next three hours, I test my driving against the vagaries of gravel groynes, errant camber, on-road bulls (Aberdeen Angus), potholes, bone-shuddering cattle grids, bends that suddenly take me headlong into glare or into blinding clouds of raised dust. All of these are taken at the highest prudent speed and with remarkable good humour on the part of my passengers.

The grader has been on the track recently, improving and levelling it. As I approach a bend, I narrowly keep my wheels away from fresh gravel, heaped up by the grader. I recall a friend and adventurer, Steve Watkins, who, blinded by the setting sun, drove his 4WD into gravel on a bend like this in the East Kimberley, and overturned. He fractured his femur in the accident and as he lay there in his vehicle, some fat from the marrow of his broken bone was released into his circulation and lodged in his brain. Steve died there alone, of the resulting stroke.

While I drive the troopie, Elijah drives Anthony crazy, constantly informing him of his satanic mission, constantly testing him with suggestions that the two swap positions.

Stolid, patient, ever firm, Anthony plays a straight bat and waits for the tablets to bite.

After fifty kilometres, Ezekiel wants to take a leak. (Much more genteel than that, he politely asks me to stop so he can go to the toilet. But the nearest toilet is back in Balgo.) Stops such as this present a fault line for the pressure of impulse within Elijah. But he misses his chance and we drive on.

Fifteen minutes later, Elijah interrupts the flow of his utterance to Anthony and directs a request to me for a toilet stop. I'd prefer not to stop, so I say, 'Not yet, Elijah. Hang on a few minutes.'

This is at 3.20 p.m.

Five minutes later Elijah is asleep, and he remains asleep until well after we pull up at Halls Creek Hospital at 6.00 p.m.

The remainder is just a drive on a tricky track through unfamiliar country with one sleeping patient and three waking blokes, one a gentle giant Pom, the second a quiet Oldest Australian, the third a middle-aged Jewish city slicker. The afternoon shines, the desert shows us her various complexions and the sun sets just as the track turns due west. Blinded, we crawl for a while, then as day fades into dusk, we play chicken with the kangaroos.

It is all pretty much uneventful, except for the moments when we hit a hidden pothole hard. Twice this happens and twice our largest passenger crashes hard against the steel roof. He grunts and rubs the sore bit for a while. When we get out, Anthony says, 'You owe me a couple of Panadol tablets, Doc.'

As I believed, we all are received at Halls Creek Hospital. With difficulty, we arouse Elijah and I wheel him into the place where I hope he will begin to heal.

Anthony gets his two Panadols, and as he drops me off at my house he says, 'I'm going straight back to Balgo' – good news for the CEO of Balgo Health. 'There are a couple of cars I noticed on the track that I'm interested in. I expect to arrest them. I know those cars, I know what they have aboard, and where they'll wait outside Balgo for the handover.'

He is referring to the booze and ganja entrepreneurs, responding to the imperative of the market: supply must rise to meet demand. One of the importers is a white man, a frequent visitor, the other indigenous, a local.

'Will you have a feed first?' I ask.

'No, a cuppa will do me, then straight back to Balgo.'

We shake hands.

◎◎◎

One hour later, I am eating some aged leftovers in my house when the phone rings. It is the nurse at Halls Creek Hospital: 'Elijah went out for a smoke and absconded.'

I am not surprised, almost relieved.

I laugh, a deep, long, full laugh. You have to laugh if you don't want to cry.

Over the next two days, Elijah and the doctors and the nurses and the police stage a re-run of our short saga in Balgo. The other players are Elijah's Halls Creek cousins. These too are the salt of the earth, endlessly concerned and patient. One, a young mother called Juanita, says, 'He wasn't always like this. It's only since he's been on the grog and those drugs.'

'What drugs, exactly, Juanita?'

'Well, now the people who bring in the drugs are mixing the ganja with ice. It's much more dangerous …'

◎◎◎

On Elijah's third day in Halls Creek, The Royal Flying Doctor Service flies him to Graylands Psychiatric Hospital in Perth, where he will be admitted as an involuntary patient. He has a drip in a vein on the back of each forearm, a catheter up his urethra and a mesh of manacles on his limbs. He is unaware of these details. Deeply sedated, his Committal Certificates at his bedside, Satan's boss sleeps.

I visit Elijah to say goodbye. The nurse has a cheering story: 'Last night he woke up, asked for a smoke, then undid his restraints and ran away again. The police brought him back, we fed him and sedated him and he agreed to get back into bed.'

It is Sunday, seven days since I first met Elijah, seven days since Supply met Demand at the Balgo sports carnival.

◉◉◉

Postscript to a love story: my wife received the email and loved the painting. It hangs now at our home.

9. WEEPING AT ONE ARM POINT

A blistering day in the Kimberley. It's a very short walk from the airconditioned clinic to the old lady's house, perhaps thirty metres, but as we step outside the heat belts me. Straight away sweat runs and my fresh shirt becomes a wet flag.

Craig is the nurse at this small clinic. I am following him on a routine house call. We are going to see Mabel, an old lady who has long been too infirm to come to the clinic.

We knock and when there is no answer, Craig pushes open the front door and announces us. We go inside, into the gloom. The air in the room is hot and still. Curtains drooping from a pelmet block most of the sunlight and trap the heat. The room is almost empty. Only a single black steel chair and a sagging stretcher bed – and silence – inhabit the room.

Stray shafts of light blind me at first. After a while I can make out a large form lying upon the broken bed. We approach. Craig speaks and Mabel opens her eyes and looks in the general direction of Craig's voice.

'How are you today, Mabel?'

A husky exhalation that sounds like, 'Who are you?'

'It's Nurse Craig, and I've got the doctor with me. We've come to check on you, Mabel.'

Mabel says nothing further. I can make out that she is old,

probably blind, very feeble, breathless, and largely helpless. A young woman – a granddaughter, a great-granddaughter perhaps – appears and we question her. No, Mabel hasn't moved from her bed today. She barely nibbled at her vegemite sandwich …

I look from the slender young woman to the leviathan form on the bed. The tasks of caring are far beyond the possible. The young woman's responses to our clinical questioning – blank, emotionally empty, inconsequential – signal no protest, no demand, no expectation.

I don't know this old lady or her history. I know only that she needs help and we cannot give it under this roof. Craig has come to the same conclusion. We hurry back to the clinic and return with the ambulance.

Fifteen minutes later, Mabel is lying on the bed in the clinic's treatment room. As I watch Mabel stops breathing. I check for a pulse; there is none, and I can hear no heart sounds.

Abruptly the slow, hot Kimberley day speeds up. Craig dives into a corner and lugs a resuscitation trolley over to the bed where Mabel lies. A pale spare woman of middle years strides into the room, pulls out an airway, a mask and an oxygen bottle.

Craig raises his right palm high then brings it down with a mighty slap onto the centre of Mabel's chest. Nothing happens.

Quickly, I place the heels of my hands on Mabel's sternum, and push forcibly downwards. *Pump! Pump! Pump! Pump! Pump!* Now the tall thin nurse squeezes a bladderful of oxygen into the airway, then it's my turn to compress the heart again, another five rib-cracking pumps.

By my reckoning, Mabel was without circulation and respiration for only three minutes – a readily survivable interval. But what other organs have been damaged previously? If we do somehow manage to salvage Mabel, will she thank us, I wonder?

But there is no time to wonder at present. Craig has an ECG monitor running and it shows no spontaneous cardiac activity, only the artificial contractions contrived by my brutality. Now Craig manoeuvres an IV drip towards where the arm veins should be. These are invisible, buried in Mabel's fatty tissue and collapsed by cardiogenic shock. Craig bends forward a long minute as he probes delicately, his face furrowed, while we 'resuscitators' bounce the large frame up and down on the bed.

Craig straightens: 'We're in.'

Now he injects adrenaline through the drip into Mabel's vein. We pump and inflate furiously to speed the drug forward to the heart.

Another hard look at the screen. We stay our fists and bladder and stare, panting and sweating; a flat line stretches from Mabel to eternity. A second dose of adrenaline, and Mabel's heart remains still.

Craig holds electric paddles at the ready. We stand back as the paddles bounce Mabel into the air and back onto the bed. The electrocardiograph is unbending. Again Craig shocks her, then a third time. No response.

As the nurse and I resume our labours, Craig draws up some atropine and injects it. I consult my watch; we have been working on Mabel for twenty-eight minutes. After thirty minutes we might in good conscience desist.

The atropine does not work. Two middle-aged people resume their exertions over an old lady's dead body as Craig asks, 'How long have we been going? Has she had her half hour?'

'Not quite,' I say and we fall to our labours again as Craig tries a final additional dose of atropine.

Then we stop.

And I exclaim, 'Look at the monitor!'

There is a heartbeat, a nice rhythm, a reasonable rate, a viable, autonomous cardiac function.

I don't know what to feel. Other than knackered and drenched … and confused. I look up and realise that my opposite number and I haven't been introduced. We shake hands. Her name is Irene.

Mabel survives for a further four minutes before her heart stops beating for good. I stand back, no longer confused.

◎◎◎

Mabel has a large family. They have been gathering outside the clinic while we were playing out our drama inside. I make my way outside. There are people everywhere and some are crossing the grass while more flow along the red sandy tracks to the clinic. Toyotas full of people are pulling up on the grass as others set off to fetch significant family members from outstations.

Searching a roiling mass of people, I come across three women seated on a low bench, their bodies entwined with others who sit at their sides and at their feet. These three sit at the kernel of tension and grief. I am sure they are Mabel's daughters. I give them the news that isn't news. My voice is broken of all knowing, all pride and power. They look up at this greybeard and they know without listening.

Quickly, soundlessly, three middle-aged women rise and flow to the door of the clinic and disappear within. Then a mighty sound rises from the treatment room, huge, gasping shrieks as of disbelief or unbearable pain. As the daughters' daughters follow, and other women follow them into the house of death, the screaming swells to a roaring.

They cry with this energy for a long time. I start to wonder that their voices don't simply wear out. But the waves of lamentation rise and rise. Then they fall away. About thirty minutes have passed.

◎◎◎

I sit outside in the shade as the day cools and dies. Across from me, sitting on the green grass facing the clinic, is a tall angular old man whom I treated this morning. I recall his visit and it comes to me that he and Mabel share a surname. And Mabel's daughters have the same lean angularity.

It turns out that that the tall man and the fat lady were once married. They have been estranged now for some time. He keeps his distance from his wife and their daughters. Separate from that clustering crowd, he sits alone, his face unreadable.

The wall of wailing has fallen, the women have gone. Now, in quietness, the leading men gather in the clinic. Their faces inward, they aggregate around the body on the bed in the centre of the treatment room. Seated, these are large men, substantial. A silent mass of humanity, they sit like a stone raised for the dead.

Much later I retrieve my possessions from the clinic and leave. As I pass, the treatment room is in silence, deserted now, except for a tall thin man bent over a mound on the bed.

10. JONATHAN'S COUNTRY

I am sitting in the cabin of a small Cessna, eight thousand feet above the Central Desert. We are flying from the tri-state border of Western Australia, South Australia and the Northern Territory. Aboard with me are Tony the pilot, who sits up front, and Jonathan who sits at my side.

Jonathan's granddaughter brought him into the clinic this morning saying, 'He's sick.' She said her grandfather had a bad cough and he couldn't breathe. Jonathan was aged and thin. He sat without speaking but his chest expressed itself audibly enough. Bent forward, he simply sat and worked hard at breathing. I listened to his lungs and the sound I heard was like the sad music of an Argentine *bandonion, a* squeezebox without a single cheerful note.

The nurse told me Jonathan came in a couple of days ago, coughing and short of breath. He was worse today despite the powerful antibiotic he had received.

We treated Jonathan with a nebuliser and a mask, but it did no good. He kept on wheezing and coughing and working hard for his breath. His coughing was punctuated by a harsh grunting sound. I listened and watched; he was excavating for sputum.

This was pneumonia. I studied his medical file: Jonathan had bronchiectasis which had completely destroyed his right lung. He had chronic fibrillation of his heart, cataracts and trachoma; and once he nearly died when his blood ran low on sodium.

The most striking thing on his medical file was a non-medical datum – his date of birth. This man was sixty-one years of age. I looked across the waiting room towards my father, who was visiting these lands with me. Dad was ninety years old and he was fitter than Jonathan.

Jonathan looked crook. Time was passing and he was not getting any better. My plane was due to leave shortly for Alice Springs, which was 900 kilometres away – a flight of two and a half hours.

Jonathan needed to be in hospital – *now*. The nurse phoned the pilot; no, there were no seats free on this afternoon's mail plane.

I wondered about the Flying Doctor, but it would take them three to six hours to get here from Kalgoorlie – if they were available; sometimes when you call them, they can't come until tomorrow because they are saving someone else today.

I rang Alice Springs Hospital and spoke to the doctor. He sounded African. I guessed he might have been in Australia for about five minutes, and had been a doctor for ten. But he listened to my story and said yes, they'd take him. This took one phone call and three minutes. In Melbourne I would spend longer than that on hold, and I would not be able to extract a promise of admission at all.

It was decision time. I didn't know what sacred protocols of medical evacuation might apply to such situations. I didn't really want to know.

I asked Jonathan whether he was willing to go to hospital in Alice. He nodded. We drove him to his home to tell his family. There they all were, four generations sitting outside on the ground. I recognised one of them, the tall slim footballer whose twisted ankle I had treated at the beginning of this morning's clinic. That young man had an easy gracefulness. At rest he was lithe, a javelin poised for the moment of flight.

And his sister was the granddaughter who brought Jonathan

to see me. She wanted to come with Grandfather, to keep him company and to look after him. There was no room, was the answer – which was nearly true.

Here were his brother, incalculably aged, and his daughter, enigmatic and taciturn. They looked up at Jonathan sitting in the cabin of the 4WD. They looked long at the old man, but there were no words.

We drove Jonathan away from his family, away from his place, without further ceremony.

Jonathan wore shorts and a t-shirt. He carried nothing – nothing but his country. He carried a lot of his country; it was caked upon his clothes and embedded in the soles of his feet and in the palms of his hands. The rest of his skin was clean, groomed with goanna oil.

The nurse drove the half-kilometre to the airfield very gently. We had aboard precious cargo, a person who, once gone, could not be replaced. For Jonathan was of the generation of first contact. Jonathan was one of a unique group – the only Australians never to have left their ancestral place.

When explorers found Jonathan's lands, they were just too remote and too dry for farming, and the prospectors never found a valuable enough resource, so no one ever drove his people away.

Until fifty years ago, whitefellas stayed away, and the children were not stolen. When they 'came in' from the desert in the 1950s and 60s, Jonathan was among them.

He would have been a teenager when he came in to this small community that whitefellas built on his lands, and they welcomed him with new diseases, like measles. It was the measles that made Jonathan cough. He coughed so hard he destroyed the elasticity of his right main bronchial tube. This was the bronchiectasis that led to the utter destruction, over years, of an entire lung.

We got Jonathan onto the plane to fly him to Alice. When he coughed up sputum, it came in green gushes and it came too fast for his old limbs and his bad eyes to catch. It went in whatever direction Jonathan was facing at the time.

I had my misgivings about this flight, not all of them merely aesthetic; we carried none of the gear of an air ambulance, the thin air at altitude could not help Jonathan's breathing, and it could make him bust a lung. I had no way of knowing whether the plane's oxygen mask would be adequate in an emergency. It was a long time since I last resuscitated anyone. What would I do, how would I feel, how well would I manage if I needed to give Jonathan mouth-to-mouth?

☉☉☉

Jonathan and I sit next to each other on the plane. Although a tall man, he is a foetus at my side, spine curled, neck flexed, his face towards the cabin floor before him. Only inches from me is his head, a rich savannah of silver hair, locks falling in crazy luxuriance, a Central Desert painting of near-concentric curves. Such vivid hair!

He sits with legs akimbo, the preferred seat of his people. Given the choice, his people generally sit upon the earth, their hips splayed. It is a stable and comfortable way of sitting.

On this plane, Jonathan's left knee is thrust outwards and presses against my leg throughout. From time to time he coughs and grunts. I reach for the tissues and place some in his hands. Useless. A direct hit on the floor in front of him.

In the desert you could spit for an eternity and never offend.

Next cough-and-grunt I am ready with a sheaf of tissues, held like a catcher's mitt. I keep my eye on the play. Cough comes to crescendo. Proffering tissues I lean across to my right at the precise moment that Jonathan turns towards me. The tissues catch a little, while Jonathan and I catch equal, larger amounts of loose chartreuse mucus. It is plentiful and very warm on the bare skin of my forearm.

Somehow mere mucus on my arm isn't a problem. Jonathan's breathing is my problem, and his – he cannot get his breath.

I look at Jonathan and picture him as a youth. The picture is very clear in the eye of my mind. I see a tall athlete, thin as a whip, erect, graceful. The picture is clear because I saw him in the person of his grandson just this morning.

That boy remains in his country while Jonathan flies 900 kilometres from his place. He flies with closed eyes – even if he were to open them he would not see these alien lands below. Those eyes don't work any more.

The Cessna can seat four. There remains one seat unoccupied. I am sorry we did not bring Jonathan's granddaughter with us. There was room for her. She would have been his eyes.

The flight is turbulent. Jonathan's light frame bounces around and more mucus is loosened. Better out than in, it emerges like a volley of buckshot. Again, some of it misses us. You would not want to be doing this work for the glamour.

It occurs to me that all of our doctoring might be irrelevant, that we might be too late – too late for Jonathan, too late for his people. Perhaps Jonathan might have waited for the Royal Flying Doctor Service to evacuate him. I cannot know whether further delay would hurt, but I think we owe him this first chance, his best chance – it is slim enough.

We are approaching Alice Springs. My ears block up as we descend. There on our left is a cleared patch with white cylindrical structures arising priapically from the desert floor. Exotic growths, they are foreign to this landscape. I ask the pilot about this modernistic installation.

'Pine Gap,' he says.

I recognise a feeling of resentment. What are they doing here in this place, in Australia? They are not here for my sake, not with my consent, nor even with my understanding. What harm might they bring into this innocent land? This is our place, piss off!

The sounds of grunting preliminaries on my right bring me back to Jonathan. I think of our presence on *his* lands and start to wonder how he feels.

It is all a bit late, and it might be irrelevant, but I want to tell Jonathan I am sorry – sorry for Pine Gap, sorry for a thousand invasions and infections, sorry for a heart too small to accommodate a granddaughter.

An ambulance taxis onto the runway as we land. Gentle medics bear Jonathan away.

They cannot know his stories. He disappears into the medical system. I track him down and follow his story for a while. But back in Melbourne a week later, when I phone the hospital they tell me they have no one by his name. They check their records then put me through to a nurse.

She says, 'Jonathan has gone.'

I hold the phone, lost for words.

The nurse says, 'Jonathan's gone. He left this morning. He's on the Cessna at this moment … Jonathan's going home to his own country.'

11. THE MAN WHO DID NOT HANG HIMSELF

The man who did not hang himself is twenty-eight years old. He has three children and a pregnant wife who is drinking right through her pregnancy. Never mind that the Intervention restricts and controls the flow of alcohol, diverting it from those at risk. There are plenty of good souls with grog permits who buy up big then triple the price and sell to those who are denied their drinking rights. The wife of the man who did not hang himself has met such a benefactor.

The man who did not hang himself takes his three children and cares for them. He sees their mother drunk, and drunk again. He looks at her pregnant belly and he sees another baby, his cousin's, born three years ago after nine months on the grog. That child looked funny from the first. The child still cannot walk or talk or hear …

The man who did not hang himself knows many who have. Too many, a couple every month, all of them young.

The Day of the Prime Minister is a day of pride; the people paint themselves and they dance and they speak to the bosses of Australia who make promises and have their photographs taken with the children. The man's youngest child, the little girl, climbs up onto the lap of the lady Minister for cuddles. The newspaper takes a photo of a cute child and a lady who looks delighted and surprised.

The man sees only a child who has no mothering.

The Night of the Prime Minister, a young dancer drinks alcohol provided by a person who has a grog permit, who is large with self-satisfaction following a highly satisfactory day. The dancing man has never had a mental illness. Only when drunk does he become violent.

That night, the young dancing man drinks, fights with his young wife. She too has been drinking. The man stabs her many, many times. She falls, apparently dead. The violent young man goes into the bush with a rope and he hangs himself.

The young woman survives.

Now she faces a new danger: her husband has died following a fight between them. She hears that his clan elders deem her culpable in his death, and decide she must face the death penalty.

She can never return to her husband's camp or clan. She must flee to refuge on the remotest island of her own clan.

The horror and the *shame* of the hanging spread in an epidemic of nausea. The man who did not hang himself is haunted by images – not of the hanging, but of the butchering. He himself has butchered game after hunting.

He sees a butchered woman, sees her flesh slashed and hacked. He sees flesh on the limbs of a living woman now as meat, chopped, minced, mashed, bloodied.

He cannot, at these moments, see his children.

The man who did not hang himself sits and weeps. His sister sees him as he gets up and goes outside. He takes a rope and he walks into the bush, still weeping. He finds a tree and throws the rope over a limb. Blinded by his tears, he throws poorly. It takes him several tries before he gets it right. By now, his sister, who has followed him, has seen and intervenes.

The family takes the man who did not hang himself to the hospital. He tells his family he does not wish to die, he just wants to clear his mind. He needs to shed the pain that drove him into the night with a rope.

◉◉◉

The man who has not hanged himself yet does not stay in hospital long. He absconds and goes back to his children.

12. ROARING MAN

Inside casualty and in the waiting area outside, there are Yolngu who sit quietly and stoically. You cannot tell from their demeanour who of them is the patient, suffering undemonstratively, and who is the companion. Inside this lagoon of resigned calm, we work and concentrate.

Abruptly, the calm is shaken by shouting and a thumping, punctuated by loud, roaring breathing sounds.

The person making the noise is a large fair man, stout and powerfully built. The lanky nurse who hurries to help him is flung about on his waving arm like an airborne crutch.

Unlike the Yolngu, this man is assertive, aggressive in fact. Shouting, he demands help: 'I'm in pain! GIVE ME SOMETHING FOR MY PAIN!'

The male nurse shows him to a cubicle. He asks, 'Where is your pain?' Large man brushes him away with a sideways thrust of his forearm; nurse stumbles backwards. 'YOU'RE A BLOODY NURSE! GET ME THE BLOODY DOCTOR!'

I step forward. 'I am the bloody doctor.' I ask, 'Where is the pain? What sort of pain is it? When did it start …?'

'IT'S HERE! IT'S IN MY BLOODY CHEST! JUST GIVE ME A SHOT!'

The bloody doctor has more bloody questions. He makes it clear there will be no treatment until the large man yields some history. At length, with exceeding ill grace, the man gives grunting monosyllables in response.

He is pale, breathing fast, gasping and sweating, his lips blueish. He moans between grunts. He is certainly in pain.

Yes, he does smoke! Yes he does have a cough – always has had! No, the pain just started, suddenly, severely. 'No it doesn't go down my arm, nor my throat, nor my back – NOT ANYBLOODYWHERE BUT MY CHEST! GIVE ME A SHOT! NOW!'

We do that, give him oxygen, insert an intravenous line and take an ECG tracing, then send him for an immediate chest x-ray. Is this a burst lung, or an inflamed membrane around the heart or a heart attack?

The ECG shows right heart strain; the chest x-ray shows an opaque area. This points to a pulmonary embolus, a blood clot blocking the artery to the lungs. It's a life and death condition anywhere. Out here in the bush, we GPs do not open the chest to remove blood clots. The man needs to be flown out by the Flying Doctors. The Darwin doctors will have to make that life and death call.

Complicated computation of arterial blood gas results, troponin tests for a possible heart attack, numerous phone calls to the air medical service, all take time. The Flying Doctors need to know, are we sending this aggressive man for a mental illness or for a physical one? If the former, we'll have to disable him chemically and physically before they'll take him.

I have no wish to tangle with this gentleman. For some reason I recall the difficulty experienced by Rasputin's assassins when they wished to subdue him.

After some negotiation, we agree it's a physical illness in a person who's a bit difficult.

The pain killers relieve his pain somewhat, but briefly. Taking blood from an artery does not sweeten our patient's disposition. He is angry again, roaring now, demanding another doctor: 'GET

ME A DOC WHO KNOWS WHAT HE'S DOING!'

In fact there are three doctors who are treating him. He waves his arms around, an angry windmill. He will not lie down. 'LYING FLAT MAKES THE FUCKING PAIN WORSE, YOU FUCKING PRICKS!'

Standing at the bedside, I see his arms are as thick as my thighs. This man is intimidating. He alarms me.

A fourth person materialises, the hospital porter, who is just as muscular as our patient. Stocky but not fat, he puts his face in the patient's and he speaks: 'Settle down, Herman. Just settle.' The porter's speech is not loud, but clear. Herman subsides.

I know the porter. His name is Robert. Like our patient, he grew up here and went to school here. He tells me that he and Herman were in the same class at school.

He and Herman understand each other; in the hospital, the porter is also Security. Herman will behave for Robert, or the Police will assist. Herman and the Police know each other very well indeed. Herman does not wish to get to know them any better.

A second, massive shot of a narcotic painkiller and Herman is snoring, a mountain on a hospital trolley, a volcano between eruptions.

While we are waiting for the plane to arrive or for Mount Herman to explode again, Robert is free to give me some background: 'Herman smokes, but I mean heavy.'

'How many a day?' I ask.

'It's not just how many, but what he smokes. It's choof mostly. Has been since he was ten. We all tried ciggies in fourth grade, and choof as well. But Herman never stopped. Joints, then bongs, and ciggies; always choof or smokes. Never see him without one or the other.'

I try to reckon up the accumulated harm; for almost three decades Herman has sucked hot, noxious gases into his lungs for most of every waking hour. This is heavy, heavy smoking. And the mixture of marijuana and tobacco is far more corrosive than the tobacco alone.

Robert continues, 'They reckon it's the choof that made him schizophrenic. Him and his brother. Herman's actually the easier of the two to handle. Choof has turned a lot of people here schizophrenic.'

'So Herman's a Yolngu?'

'Yeah.'

◎◎◎

The hospital in Darwin calls us the next day. They've done CT scans and there is indeed a pulmonary embolus. They won't be operating to remove it; they'll try drugs instead.

An operation would kill Herman: his lungs have been materially destroyed. He needs a lung transplant. He'll die if he doesn't have the transplant in the near future.

Herman is thirty-seven years old.

13. NEXT DOOR TO PARADISE

I fly to Elcho Island just offshore from East Arnhem Land, where they have no permanent doctor. The nearest hospital is forty minutes away by plane, in the great city of Gove (pop. 4000). Pretty clearly the 2600 souls on this island need a doctor, and at this moment, I am all they have.

Baby Blue

On my first morning, the health worker asks me to see a one-year-old baby. I check his date of birth: he was born a few days after my grandson Noah. He weighs just over six kilograms, a little less than half of Noah's weight. He has fallen off the bottom of his growth chart. The little boy, Jason, has a fever and he cannot breathe. He coughs, cries, then suckles for comfort. His mother's breasts are dry and Jason is dehydrated.

I look hard at Jason. He is battling mightily for air. He takes eighty-eight breaths in a minute – I count them – where twenty or so should do.

I look at Jason's darkish lips and I cannot tell whether they are usually blue like this. His nostrils flare like a racehorse's and as his ribcage expands and contracts, his muscles are sucked inwards with each breath.

Back in the city, I might feel less fearful for a child with a chest infection, but this baby has additional problems – malnutrition and anaemia, skin sores and hookworms. His resistance is compromised: this is a pneumonia, maybe septicaemia too.

Initially I am alone with Jason and his mum. Mum is a tall, slim young lady. I ask her if Jason is her first baby.

'No. Number three.'

Abruptly, she gets up and leaves the room. When she returns, she smells strongly of tobacco smoke.

I spend the morning with Jason, doing things that I do not usually do. Jason needs oxygen. I scrabble around in cupboards and drawers for the plastic tubing that will deliver oxygen to a small baby through little nasal probes. I fit this and insert the probes into Jason's nostrils. He resents this and pulls them out. I put them back in and secure them, then search for the minute gadget that will gently pinch his fingertip and measure his body's oxygen levels. I apply the gadget and take the readings. Initially they are awful: 60 per cent saturation. An alarm goes off and I jump. Then the machine completes its booting cycle, and the level rises until it reads 99.4 per cent and it stays there. A sort of reprieve.

Whenever I need to find a piece of equipment or to check on the clinic's procedure, I dash from casualty to the office of my boss, Beryl. Beryl is the Director of the Nalkanbuy clinic. She is a nursing sister with both clinical and managerial responsibilities. When I have made the ten-yard dash about ten times within an hour, Beryl decides that I need her to manage me. From now on we care for Jason together.

Beryl directs me to organise Jason's air retrieval to Gove, while she conducts a searching interview with Jason's mother. To do this I must phone the District Medical Officer. The DMO is a potentate of the remote health system. This doctor is both a gatekeeper to the local hospital and in charge of the local air medicine service.

In Melbourne it is very difficult for a GP to arrange an acute hospital admission. The Admitting Officer might agree to see and assess the patient in the emergency department, but generally baulks at an undertaking to admit. I think the assumption is that the GP is just a GP and not an expert in emergency medicine.

Outback, the GP has greater credibility. In fact, this applies equally to the Remote Health Nurse. Whenever a nurse or a doctor calls, we are signifying that we need help, and the DMO ensures we get it. And on the island, we call often; there are evacuations by air every week.

The doctor who answers my call has a soft musical voice. His accent is African and his name is Samuel. Samuel asks me a few questions, listens attentively to my answers and quickly says, 'That baby will soon be exhausted – and your clinic will be too. We'll fly in and get him. We can get a plane to you by 1330 hours. Do you think he needs a doctor aboard, or will a flight nurse be sufficient?'

We think a nurse alone will do.

It is now 10.30 a.m. and we have been working on Jason for about two hours. Samuel was sounding me out to assess our morale and our reserves of confidence. His response is adroit and tactful.

I measure oxygen saturations and chart them while Beryl battles to get fluid into Jason. She sets up all the tubing and syringes and the adhesive tape and bags of fluid that she will use for an IV drip. I hold a small arm immobile while Beryl probes a tiny vein – which is quite invisible under the dark skin – with a fine sterile needle. She says, 'I'll make one attempt at this vein – one only. I don't want to ruin a whole lot of veins for the people in Gove if I fail.'

Beryl reckons she's found the linear course of the vein. Gently she manoeuvres the needle, upwards and inwards. Gently, she sucks back with a syringe; if we have a vein, the nozzle of the syringe will fill with blood. Beryl sucks, I hold an arm thinner than my great toe, and nothing happens. Beryl tries a different angle, then another and another; no luck, a dry hole.

We have a dry baby, and no intravenous access …

The emergency room falls silent. Then Jason farts. Now a thin brown fluid issues from his lower body onto the thick cotton sheeting on the trolley. Lying on this adult-sized bed, Jason looks absurdly small, and – if you stand back from him, if you don't look too closely at his nostrils, at his rushing ribs, at his flying diaphragm – he looks adorably cute. Too small for a one-year-old, he is a doll, an imitation.

But Jason is in trouble. A couple of hours ago, he fought the oxygen probes and clung to his mother. Now he has strength only to breathe and doze. The lake of smelly fluid around him widens. He is shitting out the water of his life, and with it the sugar that is his body's fuel and the minerals that operate his muscles.

Unchecked, diarrhoea is an all-out attack of diminishment; it will eventually dry a baby out and his circulation weakens then fails. His blood sugar falls, and he may lose consciousness and start to fit; in the extreme, potassium is lost and muscles fail. No muscle function, no breathing effort, no cardiac contraction. No Jason.

Jason's mother offers him her breast. He mouths the nipple for a moment, then dozes again. His mother stands and stares at her son, then flees for another smoke.

I look at the pale brown lake and once again I feel that deep sinking fear that came often to me as a junior resident doctor, working alone at night with a failing patient. Am I going to lose him? Who will save him? Who will save *me*?

In this case, the answer is Beryl. (On first meeting her I thought: Beryl – a semi-precious stone. I have undervalued her.)

That redoubtable Beryl pulls tubing from a cupboard and a large syringe from a drawer, then grabs some oral rehydration fluid from the dispensary. She insinuates a fine tube through Jason's nostril, threading it past the oxygen probe. He gags feebly and falls still. There is a look of stern purpose on Beryl's face as she feeds the tube past unseen landmarks of internal anatomy towards Jason's stomach. She lets out her breath. 'There, that should do it.' But something is wrong – the tubing peeps out between Jason's lips. It curled in his throat and sits there mocking us. Another deep breath, another intense session, as Beryl frowns and works in slow centimetres. She straightens, watches Jason for a moment or two, then – satisfied – she swiftly fills the syringe with the rehydrating solution and squirts tentative dribbles into his stomach. Then stops and watches again. No fluid comes back.

Perhaps a tide is turning.

Meanwhile I continue to log Jason's respirations at 88 gasps per minute.

We two spend the morning working on Jason, watching and supporting and – in my case at least – silently asking him: Are you going to die this morning?

By lunchtime Jason hints that he will not die today. The nasal prongs have worked their way loose and hang at a distance from his nostrils, directing the oxygen towards his right ear at a handy four litres per minute. But his oxygen saturations have not fallen!

At lunchtime we take Jason and his mum to the airport in the ambulance – Beryl and I are the ambulance officers here – and hand him over to the flight nurse, once again feeding oxygen into his nostrils through the forked tongue of the plastic tubing.

Jason and his mum fly out to Gove. The retrieval by the local Flying Doctor Service in an aircraft equipped for all critical contingencies – complete with flight nurse – at a cost of $8000. Beryl tells me that there is an urgent retrieval from Elcho Island of this nature every 2.2 days. And many more fly out on regular flights for x-rays and scans and specialist appointments in Gove or Darwin.

A conversation has been going on, intermittently, all morning. It is a conversation between Beryl and Jason's mother. The two women know each other well; the mother is a trained health worker, until very recently employed in this Children's Clinic. The conversation (to which I do not contribute) is a painful one.

Beryl asks her former worker, 'Did you feed Jason any breakfast this morning?'

'*Yohh* – yes,' says Mum.

'What did you give him, Matala?'

'Porridge.'

'Real porridge, Matala? Not just flour in milk?'

'*Yohh*, real porridge.'

'Why is he so small, Matala?'

No answer.

'Matala, did you eat this morning?'

No answer. Matala looks down.

Beryl looks up and across the bed in the emergency room where we are spending our morning. Her eyes meet mine. There is weariness and sorrow in her face, and a deep perplexity. Her face is asking – after all these years – *why*?

For a while there is silence. Then Beryl says, in a kindly tone, 'Matala, you must be hungry. Go and get yourself some food. We'll look after Jason. Go quickly and hurry back.'

Matala goes without lingering, without farewell to Jason. All morning, she has seemed only half-engaged with him. She goes and does not soon return.

While we are alone with Jason, now a very real, very alert, hypoxic little witness to his own plight and to the struggles in the emergency room, Beryl lets out a series of long and bitter sighs. Then she gives me her reading of Matala – Matala the health worker and Matala the mother.

'She's a highly intelligent girl, highly capable. She went to Batchelor College on the mainland and she learned a lot. She became a really skilful worker, you know, accurate and sophisticated. She would have been an asset here. But she wasn't reliable. Recently, she missed more and more days. A few days ago, I told her it couldn't go on. I told her she couldn't work like this. I said not to come any more, not to come until she was ready to come to work every day.'

Matala returns in a cloud of smoke. She carries her lunch – a large bottle of Coke and a bag of hot potato chips. She sits on the floor of the emergency room and starts to eat.

Now Beryl's angst goes into overdrive.

'I know why Jason is so small, why he gets sick. I know and you know! He is small because you have no food for him. There is no food because you spend all your *rupiah* on gambling and on smokes! You have plenty *rupiah*, you have enough for food. You have Child Support, and Work For the Dole. Your husband has Unemployment Benefits. But you have no food for Jason and no food for yourself. All your *rupiah* gone, gone on cards and for smokes.'

Matala has not looked up from her chips. She has eaten little.

' When you don't eat, you don't make enough milk. *And Jason starves!*'

Matala has not looked up. Shamed, she says nothing.

I too say nothing.

After a while Beryl calms down and commands me to accompany her to her office, the old ten-yard dash, where I will write a letter of referral for Jason.

'Make sure you ask the hospital to get Children's Services onto this. That child has to be protected. His older sister had to be taken from Matala and placed in the care of her aunt, Matala's sister.'

I do as I am bid.

My mind goes back to the country town of my childhood. The year was 1953. Leeton was agog with the coronation in London of a new queen. Back home, we wouldn't count Aboriginal people in our census, nor give them the vote until nearly twenty-five years had passed. In 1953 we still took mixed-blood children from their families with the full force and authority of the law. In my hometown kindly matrons said, 'They'll be placed in a good home. *It is for their own good.*'

As I write my fateful letter now to Children's Services, I ask myself: am I helping to steal someone's child – 'for his own good'?

The local gambling schools operate around the clock. On our

79

way to the airport in the ambulance, we pass the card players sitting in a circle on the ground. Early next morning they are still there, still playing as I pass them on my early morning run. They sit gratefully under the street light that we Balanda (white people) installed for them and gamble their *rupiah* away.

Sourly, I reflect on our other gifts to the Yolngu. We taught them to smoke, we introduced them to our diseases and to money and playing cards. They are deeply in our debt.

I am starting to feel the growth of a metaphor on my upper arm. In moments of contemplation it grips me like a ghost. It is a black armband.

The Hearing

It is my final morning on the island. In my sleep overnight, I feel or hear or dream the close drone of a plane landing or taking off. In the morning, I drive to work with Mandy, the Child Health nurse, who reports on her active night on call: 'We had an evacuation last night. An old man, well, not so old really – he is only fifty-five years of age – he couldn't breathe. We gave him oxygen, put in a drip, stabilised him, then took him to the airport in the ambulance. He wasn't too bad by the time the plane arrived. Perhaps he didn't really need to go in the end. But they took him.'

At the clinic there is more news, and different. Beryl looks serious. She says quietly, 'We've had a death overnight. There will be a hearing today. The death won't be announced until then. The name of the deceased won't be spoken. Most of the family don't know yet.'

It turns out that the deceased was last night's evacuee. He was comfortable during the flight, but had a sudden cardiac arrest on descent and could not be resuscitated.

I have an unwelcome thought: was the deceased my patient? Was his death preventable? I retrieve the file and sure enough, there is my handwriting; I saw him only a few days ago. My entry closes with the note: 'Cardiac failure, respiratory failure, renal disease – needs home oxygen for palliation.'

Whatever the clinical notes might say, and irrespective of the certified cause of death, the relatives of the deceased might determine that an individual is to blame, perhaps the doctor. In that case, retribution would be mandated; law would require it.

I want to come back here again to work, but I don't want to be speared. Warily, I ask Beryl, 'What is a hearing?'

'It's a formal ceremony. People are very upset when a death occurs. They all gather to hear the death announced. It's very solemn. No one speaks aloud about the death before the hearing and, out of respect, no one will mention the name of the deceased for some time after the burial.'

'How long?' I wonder.

Beryl says, 'It depends. The family determines how long, usually not less than a year, but it varies. It can complicate our work here, because we often have two, three or more files all bearing the same name as the deceased person. Then we have to identify a person by a western name, Samuel or Britney, or whatever.'

My last clinical action in Galiwin'ku (the largest community on Elcho Island) is to write the death certificate of an old man, a cripple who dies at fifty-five, five years younger than I am.

Before that, I walk up to the store for a final purchase. I want to buy a lap-lap, a souvenir of the colourful fabrics that decorate the stately people of this island. But the store is closed. The takeaways are closed. For the first time in my sixteen days in Galiwin'ku, you cannot buy junk food. There is a tide of people flowing from the direction of the clinic, from the houses, up from the shore, flowing, wave upon silent wave, all flowing across the town to somewhere not known to me, known to the people, somewhere where they'll attend the ceremony of the hearing, somewhere where a person with a name that will not soon be again heard will be sent on his long journey.

And after only half an hour, the town is alive again, store and Council open. There is movement, sick people come to the clinic, healthy kids come for dental checkups, laughing babies come, receive their shots, cry lustily and submit to the pacifying flow of mother's milk.

The Women's Health nurse, Kelly, tells me more about the observance of a death. 'When an old person passes away, everyone is very sad. The older the person, the greater the grief, the more prolonged the sorry business. That person was tied to people by many years of connection and memory of event and loss. More time, more ties, more pain.'

Every ancient who *passes* or is *lost* – those gentle old-fashioned euphemisms – every old person takes with them some memory, some history, something the community will lack and that will not be again.

Stoning Bimini

There is a tall young woman who frequents the clinic. I see her in the office, on the verandas, in and out of the consulting rooms. She clocks on in the mornings and again after lunch, as the other workers do. It isn't clear to me what she does in the clinic or which section she belongs to. She moves around a lot, and sometimes you can hear her approach, chattering in a fluent bird-like stream of soft sound. Then she is in my room, in my face, writing words without apparent meaning in heavy blue crayon on the medical file that lies open on my desk. Her name is Bimini.

Late on a Sunday afternoon, I bump into her in the street. She walks up to me, keeps coming, comes to a stop at a breath's distance and speaks into my face: 'Will you buy a drink for me?'

The request is unexpected. I can't think of a reason not to do so, so I buy Bimini a bottle of fruit juice.

Eventually a nurse tells me, 'Bimini has chronic schizophrenia, and her medication doesn't quite keep her stable.'

What is she doing in the clinic, I wonder. What is her role?

It turns out that Bimini has no official function. The clinic is her place of shelter. Elsewhere in Galiwin'ku, on the streets, in the open places, they stone her. She clocks on and clocks off here, and she feels she belongs.

Singing me home

It is my last morning on the island. I have been a visiting doctor in Aboriginal communities in many different parts of the country, but it is only here that I start to feel I could be something more than a medical tourist. Walking into the clinic this morning, I fell into step with Rachel, one of the health workers. Rachel said, 'You are flying out today?'

'Yes.'

'Will you come back? We want you here. You are a good doctor.'

I am aware that people here seem more comfortable talking with me than others in other places, in past years. I have no illusions that I am a better doctor; it a simple matter of the eclipse of the last remaining black hairs on my head and in my beard. The Yolngu look at my silver hair and my wrinkled face and they see an elder. And they give me at last a sense that I might be useful. As well as this, they give me a reminder of my own absurdity, of the absurdity of expecting to comprehend a people, a culture, an island, far, far from my own.

Every morning there is a meeting of all the clinic staff. The bureaucrats here love meetings. I think they are addicted to them. All of us, Yolngu and Balanda, come to the meeting. We sit down on the ground or lounge around in the bright morning sunshine while Cherryl tells us the news – who is flying in today, who is flying out, who is here, who is away, who just can't be found at the moment.

Before this last meeting I whisper to Cherryl, 'I'm flying out today. I'd like to say something – a goodbye and a thank you – after the meeting.' She nods and grins slyly.

We all gather in the sun or out of it on the veranda. Cherryl speaks: 'Howard wants to say something.'

I protest: 'I'll wait until you've finished with all the other clinic business.'

'There is no other business today. It's your turn.'

These days on Elcho Island have felt highly significant. Although I comprehend little of what has passed these two weeks and two days, I am certain of the way the people affect me. I feel an irresistible liking for the Yolngu and a great respect. In such a short space, I suppose I can't have formed affections so deep that I'll feel grief on leaving, but there is something, something real.

I look around me at my colleagues seated in clusters, some on the grass, some on the veranda. There they all are, in the blaze of morning light, or dark in the deep shade. I take in the faces and the forms of my days here. I take out the scrap of paper upon which the teacher at the school has written the words I want to say in Yolngu Matha.

I feel their bulk and taste their chalky unfamiliarity in my mouth as I read them aloud. After a couple of lines, I look up and pause. Is this okay? Is my gesture misfiring, do the people find this disrespectful, mocking even?

But the Yolngu are nodding, encouraging me. I hear *yohh*, *yohh*, from smiling faces to my right and to my left. I read on and get to the finish. Everyone is smiling.

For no clear reason I decide I will sing. 'This is a song in Hebrew – it is a song of the people of my tribe.' I close my eyes and start to sing:

> All of the world,
> The entire world,
> Is a very narrow bridge,
> A very narrow bridge.
> But the main thing …

I can hear a sweet sound, a high voice swelling, rising above mine, keeping time. I stop singing and listen. Someone *is* singing, a woman. I look around and it is Bimini who is singing, poor mad Bimini, singing with a purity and a sweetness that leave me amazed. Rapt, I listen. But the health workers shush Bimini. They round on her, tell her to be quiet. After a while, Bimini does fall silent. They have killed my mockingbird.

I resume:

> But the main thing
> The principal thing
> Is not to fear …

Bimini is singing again, people are shushing, but she sings on heedless. She sits and sings, and as she sings, her tall, slim body sways with her song. And as she sways, she claps her hands in time, with slow rhythmic grace.

I have stopped singing. I sit and laugh, laugh with hilarity and laugh for joy and beauty. Soon the people, seeing me unoffended, stop shushing and start to smile, then they are laughing too. And Bimini pours out her soul in ecstasy. When at length she finishes, we all clap and her smile is a thing of beauty.

Then I finish my song:

> … not to fear at all.
> The main thing,
> The principal thing
> Is to have no fear at all.

More applause. I translate and the people nod.

I continue: 'Soon I will go back to my family, and my small grandchildren will ask me where I have been. I will say – "I have been in Galiwin'ku." Then they will ask, "What sort of place is that, *Saba*?" Then I will sing them a song about this place and about you people.'

It is a place of friendly smiles
And crocodiles;
Of barking dogs
And croaking frogs.

The song for my grandchildren goes on for a number of stanzas of similar quality. The Yolngu like them, and later, back in Melbourne, Jesse and Ellie like them too.

It is time for me to finish, to say goodbye. 'My people have a word for goodbye that also means peace, and we also use it for hello. The word is *shalom*. I am going to sing shalom, to say goodbye, and to say that I will come back and say hello again, if you will have me.'

Heveinu shalom aleichem,
Heveinu shalom Aleichem
Heveinu …

I am singing again, eyes closed, trying not to fall off the melody line, trying to reach those high notes, when I realise that another voice is singing along, singing the same words – in Hebrew! I open my eyes. This time it is not Bimini who accompanies me. She is sitting in front of me and to my left; the sound comes from my right. The singer is an old lady, Guymini, one of the Strong Women.

We sing and finish the song together.

◎◎◎

As usual, I drive another of the Strong Women, Ninnigur, home at lunchtime. She asks me to give a lift also to Guymini. Guymini sits next to me in the front of the ute, splendid beneath her crown of silver curls and in her brilliant yellow dress.

'Where did you learn that song, Guymini?'

'Jerusalem. I was in Jerusalem for four weeks a good few years ago.'

Then Guymini looks at me intently for a moment and says, 'I am going to adopt you.'

I feel as if I have been anointed.

I think of my own old mother, how she would be amused and proud.

After a bit, I say gently, 'Thank you.'

Guymini continues: 'I want you to be my father.'

PART THREE

ACCEPTANCE

And many weep for sheer acceptance, and more
Refuse to weep for fear of all acceptance

(From 'An Absolutely Ordinary Rainbow' by Les Murray)

14. AN AMBIGUOUS PARADISE

Imaginings

Elcho Island is a speck in the Arafura Sea. Before my visit to Elcho I knew nothing about it, nothing beyond the imaginings that I brought with me. I discover a paradise – a constantly shifting paradise, an ambiguous place that subverts all preconception and easy generalisation.

To get to Elcho Island from Darwin you take the Air North flight to Maningrida in an aircraft designed for hunchbacks and dwarves. At Maningrida you change to an even smaller aircraft to fly to Elcho itself.

I clamber to my seat at the back of the plane, where my neighbour is a toddler with tight black curls and a packet of chewing gum. With great seriousness, she removes a stick of gum from the pack and, concentrating intently, she peels off the wrapper and pushes an impossibly large stick of gum into her tiny pink mouth. She is a miniature, a slightly snotty cherub.

For most of this short flight her Mum, a slight young lady with lovely skin and the same tight black curls, is absorbed in some music that enters her head through earphones. Face on, Mum looks like Halle Berry.

'Are you visiting Elcho, or do you live there?' I ask.

'I live on Elcho. We've just been visiting Darwin,' she says, then adds, 'You've got to get away every so often.' She flashes me a conspirator's smile, the grin of a teenager caught wagging school. A return ticket costs plenty, so she must be pretty keen to 'get away'.

Maningrida is an outpost in Arnhem Land – on the outer edge of the edge of the Australia I know. I look about me at the rust and the glorious shabbiness of the place. The departure lounge is a shade area under a tin roof on the edge of the runway. Wild and scruffy and luxuriant, the rainforest presses irresistibly against the modest airport buildings. Kids and dogs run free between adults who are meeting travellers. There is a lot of lounging around. Are we in Africa?

I feel a bit disoriented by the heat and the disorder and disrepair, the indifference to time and to timetable. I am outside the edge of my known world.

Passengers mill in and out of the tiny airport offices. Preoccupied with my luggage and tickets and photo ID, I look for someone who will confirm that I am on the next plane. I find an informal bloke with reassuring epaulettes, who says, 'Yeah, you'll be right.' Halle Berry also wishes to confirm her flight to Elcho. She asks Mister Epaulettes whether he has her booking. He consults his passenger list and her name isn't there. Neither seems surprised. She says, 'This usually happens.' She doesn't look worried.

Standing by himself beneath the tin roof is a thin and wrinkled man, the only person here not engaged in conversation. He looks comfortable in his solitude. I ask him whether he has been to Elcho before.

'Yes', he says, 'I have been there before.'

'What do you do there?' I ask.

'I teach. I'm a relief teacher. This is the third time I've done it. It will be the last.'

His sentences emerge fully made and precise, but with such a lack of emphasis that man and utterance are almost transparent. His words trail off into inaudibility. I lean forward to hear. I ask what I am thirsting to learn: 'Is the local culture in good shape?'

'Not like it was,' he says. 'About twenty years back, when I lived on the island, there was ceremony or corroboree every night. Every night I'd fall asleep to the sounds of clapsticks and singing and stamping feet. Just occasionally, if I couldn't sleep, it would be the quietness that was keeping me awake: no ceremony, no sleep. But on my last visit, there was no corroboree in the whole six weeks.'

'Why have things changed?' I ask the teacher. 'What has made the difference?'

The teacher shrugs. He doesn't know. He screws up his lean face and interrogates the shimmering distance.

We board the very small plane for the short flight to Elcho. It is so short that the earache of our ascent merges with the earache of descent. Halle Berry's daughter, a gum-chewing prodigy, peels and ingests stick after stick of gob-stopping gum. She shows no sign of earache.

We land in Galiwin'ku, the town on Elcho Island. My house is about a hundred metres from the airstrip. There are three bed-rooms in a house that I will occupy alone. It feels a bit wasteful; perhaps they expect me to use all three rooms by turns.

There are about 2500 indigenous people on this oblong island four kilometres wide and sixty kilometres long. They call them-selves Yolngu. I am one of the hundred so people on the island who are not Yolngu. They call us Balanda.

We are here on these homelands to provide services that the people need. What value the Yolngu place on our services is not immediately clear.

It is a matter of shocking fact that some health statistics across Arnhem Land are worse now than they were thirty years ago. Three decades of our best efforts and best intentions have left people worse off. But Elcho Island is a local health showpiece. By the end of my sixteen days here, the question of our value remains moot.

I make a preliminary tour of Galiwin'ku. There are houses on short stilts, some dilapidated, some completely ruined, yet others with a tidy, suburban appearance. The little town has a sleepy Sunday afternoon feeling. Dotted here and there are low mounds of topsoil into which tall bamboo poles have been planted. On the top of each pole flies a rectangular banner of coloured cloth. The effect is like a small garden plot with blooms of bright fabric.

Each mound, I discover, is a grave. The various banners represent the respective clans on the island. On a given grave, the banner of the deceased's clan predominates. Each of the other clans plants a banner as a sign of respect.

Wherever you go in Galiwin'ku, you find these memorials where the dead lie in their own soil. Above them fly their clan's colours and between them naked children play and lazy dogs lie in the sun.

There are a couple of graves not far from the front and back doors of the clinic, and whenever I emerge I encounter these reminders of death. The effect is not morbid. More than anything, they imply a continuity between the generations and an unbordered relation between people and land.

On my first day, I walk to work. Bouncing ahead of me, a five-year-old boy dances and swings on his mother's arm as they walk along the wide shaded verandas of the clinic. Animated, exuberant, this little fellow looks like the embodiment of a bright future.

He carries something in his small hand, a DVD from the store, still in its cellophane wrapping. I read the label – *The Incredibles*. Is this, I wonder, the Yolngu future, to become just another cultural satellite of the United States?

◎◎◎

A night time at the Darwin Festival. I meander through an outdoor art show, lost in wonder at prints of etchings from Yirrkala in East Arnhem Land, floodlit and mounted on tree trunks. The winding walk across emerald lawns is punctuated by one encounter after another with beauty. The media are anything but traditional, while the content is authentically Yolngu.

Nearby is a tent city where they sell weary takeaway foods, junk crafts and grog art. But here too you can buy CDs of contemporary music from the Top End. I buy *Djarridjarri* by the Saltwater Band, a group of young musicians from Elcho Island. The cover notes list their names: Yunupingu, Dhurrkay, Garawirrtja. These names become familiar to me in my days in Galiwin'ku.

This music throbs with life, some of it imported ('We love reggae music ...'), but all of it soaked in tradition, much of it sung 'in language'. The lyrics are salted here and there with chanting by traditional elders.

I do some traditional chanting of my own. The eve of the ninth day of the Jewish month of Av finds me on Elcho Island, sitting on the hard floor, singing *Lamentations* by feeble candlelight. It is the sack and rape of Jerusalem 2000 years ago that I lament.

We have carried out this observance now for 2000 years. At the same time, elsewhere in the Jewish world – on the beaches and at the nightspots of Tel Aviv, Elwood, St Kilda – young Jews are dancing and disporting, oblivious to the traditional restrictions of these Nine Days of Mourning. Notwithstanding that obliviousness, who could doubt the continuing vitality of Jewish cultural practice and belief?

The cover notes of *Djarridjarri* carry the lines: 'Let us become one and think of our elders and follow them with our minds and our feet.'

The fifth track of the CD is the longest, and my favourite. It is called *Warwu* (Grieving). It is more a love song than a song of grief. It sings the yearning love of a people for their land. The lyrics' particularities, their exploding images, their longing for return, their free embrace of diaspora as a chosen expression of identity, all feel very familiar to the lamenting Jew who sits upon the floor. Instead of going and reclaiming our hereditary land – or as well – some sit and sing and grieve. I recall the Hassidic tale of the lost fire …

> Many generations ago there lived a great mystic Master. This man held secret knowledge of great power. From time to time, when his people were in an extremity of suffering, the Master would go deep into the forest. There, in a clearing, he would light a fire, dance, chant esoteric verses and call upon God to save His suffering people. He would return from his seclusion and the crisis was averted; the people were saved.
>
> Time and again he resorted to the isolation, the fire, the dance and secret song, and each time, salvation came to his people.
>
> In time the Master grew old and died.
>
> Another crisis arose. None of the disciples knew the ceremonial. They made their way into the forest, found the clearing and lit a fire. And they prayed: O Master of the universe, save us. Save us, even though we are unsure of what to do. We have lost the dance and the song. Save us as you saved us in the days of our Master. And the people were saved.
>
> In a later generation, the disciples had passed on. Destruction again threatened the faithful, and now with no surviving initiate, the people prayed: O Master of the universe, we have no initiated leader. No one knows the prayer or any of the secret ceremonies. We do not even know where we should light the fire. We remember only that in past times our forefathers lit fire, danced and sang and prayed and You sent salvation. O Father, pray save us again now.
>
> And once again, the people were saved.

Sometimes the act of recalling something past, of giving voice to loss is sufficient to experience identity. In a time of loss and cultural degradation, shared memory can define the group.

Is that the case among the Yolngu?

◎◎◎

On the morning of my fourteenth day on Elcho Island Kelly, the Women's Health nurse, says, 'There's going to be an initiation tonight.'

I am a *mohel*, an initiating surgeon to eight-day-old Jewish males. I am immediately curious. 'Will there be a circumcision? Can anyone go?'

The nurse is clear: 'Yes, there certainly will be a circumcision and no, we Balanda cannot go, not unless we're invited.'

I wonder aloud, 'What instrument do they use here – a razor blade?' (That's what they use – *and repeatedly re-use* – around Alice.)

'No,' says Kelly. They come to the clinic and we give them a sterile surgical blade.'

Children

Kelly looks after all the intimate aspects of women's health. Guarded by her phalanx of Strong Women, Kelly's office is around a corner, out of the way of passing foot traffic.

I am a male and I must keep my distance, culturally excluded from treating women for gynaecological problems, for pregnancy or for sexually transmitted disorders. Some females, generally old, old ladies, will consult me about matters above the belly button or below the knee.

Everywhere I look there are kids. Toddlers and babies and pre-schoolers and school-waggers, healthy kids, sick kids – kids everywhere. And everywhere, there is an older sister or cousin, mum or youthful grandma, or aunty. Kids and dogs are the small creatures that strike my newcomer's eye, the former nurtured, the latter neglected.

I ask Kelly, 'Is abortion taboo?'

'No. There are about seven or eight terminations a year.'

This doesn't seem to me to be a large number. 'So are the rest of the teenage girls happy to become mothers?'

'Yes and no. They get $4000 from the government for having a baby. $4000 is a lot of money for a teenage girl: it's enough for a plasma TV. Some kids are willing to give birth for the sake of a plasma TV.'

This takes some digesting.

I think of Nejesda, the foster-mother of four babies, the biological mother of none, who says she hungered for a baby. I wonder too what status attaches to fertility.

Kelly's answers take me at a tangent: 'There are young girls here who will give birth to a baby just so they can have something of their own, someone to love, someone to love them.'

Then, 'There are five women on the island on IVF.'

In the world outside Elcho, a short course of IVF treatment would be priced by the market alongside a plasma TV. 'Who pays for it?' I wonder.

'The women pay, their families pay. They badly want a baby.'

I see lots of women breastfeeding their babies in Galiwin'ku. Breastfeeding is the rule here, and it seems to come naturally and to go well. Mothers from the age of thirteen up, otherwise extremely shy of bodily exposure, sit or stand around in the clinic, babe at the breast, quite unembarrassed.

Lots of women shout at their children. I recoil as I hear the sound, a sort of hoarse roaring, but the child does not. Is a raised voice not an angry voice?

Kelly reminds me, 'Very many children here have chronically discharging ears. There are holes in the eardrums that do not heal. Very many children have impaired hearing as a result.' I have heard estimates that the 'very many' in fact comprise eighty per cent of the population. Deaf children become deaf adults. In the kingdom of the deaf, perhaps you have to shout simply to be heard.

I ask Kelly my key question, a clumsy one: 'What is the value here of the child?' Kelly listens and looks at me squarely then she replies, 'There are some people here who value their dogs more than their kids.'

I know that the grief is great when an old person dies. 'What about the death of a baby?'

'We had a cot death not so long ago; only the immediate family mourned. They were sad but the sorrow was not broad or deep in the community. Not like the death of an old person.'

I recall my feelings following the death of my own extremely aged father. His death was a release. At the time, I held my new grandchildren close; I was hugely sad at the loss of Dad, but I knew it wasn't a tragedy. But to lose one of our babies would be unbearable.

That thing ... you know

People do not walk about at night. There are spirits. It is foolhardy to provoke them.

A person becomes sick and the community understands that a spiritual force is at play. Perhaps the sick person has offended against the marriage laws, perhaps in some other manner. Or someone has 'sung' him in retribution for a wrong.

When the person becomes sick, the Balanda doctor offers treatment, but true cure lies in identifying the spiritual wrong and attending to it.

Here in Galiwin'ku men keep away from health matters; health concerns, clinics, health workers, the Strong Women of the Women's Health Clinic – to the men, each of these ostensible positives actually evokes the negative. They imply the opposite forces, they imply sickness, the play of a bad spirit. Men try to keep far from these concerns; they are principally a woman's affair and generally reside in women's hands.

A man will refer to the bad spirit only obliquely, preferring to avoid explicit mention of that force of ill fortune. Instead of *golka* (bad spirit), a man might click his fingers expressively, pause and say 'You know ...'

(When my late father-in-law developed the symptoms that he accurately identified as lung cancer, he said to his sister, 'I think I've got *yenne zach*', Yiddish for 'that thing', the unnameable.) Some things are literally too unlucky for words and some words are too unlucky to say.

On the other hand, there are the Strong Women!

In Galiwin'ku, the bunch of women who support Kelly in Women's Health are called the Strong Women. I write it with capitals and I see them that way. They are capital women and they do a capital job.

I try to capture with my camera the likeness of these women, their power and bearing. I fail, of course.

But my mind holds their images. Here is Bora – tall as a Somali model, graceful beyond words; here is Guymini – aged, curly-headed, vivacious; here is Ninnigur – old too, and frail and breath-less, yet unquenchably gay, earnest only about health, a leader, a role model.

The group observes an eloquent reticence. In their silence and decorum there is pride and purpose. Barefoot, they walk the verandas in quiet confidence and impregnable dignity. Various in age and in personality, these women are the community's backbone.

It is these women who give their sisters the confidence to come in and see the Balanda nurse. Shy, fearful, often ashamed, the patients come in to the clinic under the wing of the Strong Women, who interpret for them. They interpret more than mere words; they explain the entirety of an alien clinical culture that brings to their wombs the mystery of ultrasound, and to their ears the magic of the audible beating of an unborn baby's heart.

A woman's boyfriend has an STD. Somehow, discreetly, the Strong Women track down the unwitting female partner and bring her in. Shielded by the Strong Women, she receives effective, timely, confidential treatment. The Strong Women protect their sister and preserve her fertility.

In Galiwin'ku you'd have to be blind not to be a feminist.

Missionaries

I visit the church. A large weatherboard structure, it accommodates all the denominations on the island. Hand-painted sheets of fabric hang inside the door. The odd louvre is missing from the windows and the weatherboards could do with some paint.

The entire atmosphere is one of simplicity and modesty.

I step into the vestibule and peek through the doorway. The empty space is shady and restful, with shafts of light lancing across the dim interior. On a shelf in the vestibule a series of short prayers have been handwritten neatly upon cardboard placards. One prayer implores the Creator to inspire all of His children to worship Him solely as Christians.

This might imply that a person's worship might be second-rate simply if it is not Christian. But do the Yolngu take offence? How could I know if they were offended? As a people they do not seem to complain much. They seem to me to be remarkably free of anger.

I am learning here not to trust guesses and seemings, so I check out some of my surmises with the nurses: 'Yolngu feel anger as much as anyone else; if they don't show us, it's because they don't want to appear ill-mannered.'

Of a population of 2500, the Sunday congregation this week numbers fifty or so people. If only a minority of Yolngu are actively Christian, the broad community remains strongly influenced by the Mission that used to run the island. In the Mission days, there were productive industries here: forestry, fisheries and orchards. People were expected to conform to a western ethic of work, and – according to Beryl – they did so. Now those industries have withered away.

The older ladies among the Strong Women were trained on the Mission. They are leaders today.

The Mission taught and enforced the use of English. I wonder how much this was a good or a bad thing? English is a second language for many, but a third, fourth or even a fifth for others. For such a person, a conversational exchange in English might require a Yolngu to carry out four or five acts of silent translation. As a doctor I find a little English is – like a little knowledge – a dangerous thing. It carries the danger that the doctor thinks the patient is on the same wavelength, whereas in fact, translation fatigue has set in and meaning falters long before good manners fail.

The Yolngu nods 'Yohh, yohh,' and we part, marooned on opposite shores of a sea of meaning.

☉☉☉

To this day, young Balanda turn up at Elcho to do mission work, useful things. While I am in Galiwin'ku, for example, mission volunteers are sinking a well at Gawa, an outlying homeland that has no fresh water.

On a sunny Saturday morning I sit on the deck looking over my backyard and read my Sabbath prayers. In my prayer shawl and my skullcap, I am unmistakeably Jewish. When I finish, my neighbour – a teacher at the school – greets me from the other side of the fence where he is eating an outdoor breakfast. Each of us might be in heaven, so peaceful and warm is this morning.

'Shalom,' he calls. Then he speaks a few words to me in Hebrew and, pleasantly surprised, I respond in the same tongue.

'Where did you learn Hebrew?' I ask.

'*Birushalayim*' – in Jerusalem, on a study mission organised by his church on the mainland.

The local arts and crafts and the oral histories tell us of repeated contact between these islands and visitors from Indonesia. Just around the corner from the local Arts Centre, in a tidy building set in mature gardens, I find the Bible translators who are translating the Bible into Yolngu Matha.

But there are no Koran translators. From the point of view of the long history of contact with Maccassans – traders and fishers from Indonesia, an Islamic influence might be expected. Oddly there is none.

The facts?

As my sixteen day stay draws to a close, I remark to Kelly that the Yolngu here seem not to practise violence. In sixteen days, I don't see a single bashed or gashed patient. No one is drunk, no one is high or crazed on petrol. Why, I wonder.

Kelly is a straight talker and she sets me straight: 'When someone is bashed, they stay away from the clinic because they are ashamed. The people here decided they would have no petrol on the island and no alcohol. Kava is allowed. People drink kava, get drunk and fall asleep. Although chronic kava excess will eventually rot their liver or kidneys, people don't become violent with Kava.

'An occasional outboard motorboat arrives and kids milk the tank and sniff the petrol. When that happens the elders ship the sniffers out onto one of the smaller islands close by. That way, they don't influence other kids by their example.'

I chew on this, then ask, 'Am I mistaken, or is it a fact that this is a relatively healthy community?'

Kelly says, 'It is a healthy community, one of the healthier ones. The people from Menzies School of Public Health in Darwin love Galiwin'ku. They hold us up as a model for other communities. And they have the statistics that show better health – better than it used to be here, and better than other places. You are right; this is a healthier place.'

I emerge from Men's Health one morning and find a good-looking young man standing just outside. He flashes me a smile and stands there. I pass him, duck into the Beryl's office and out again, heading back to Men's Health. The young man is still there, going nowhere, still smiling.

When I emerge later, he is at a close remove. Our eyes meet and he nods. The etiquette goes something like this: I have noticed the man and he knows I have noticed him. He has not greeted me – in fact, a friend reports that there is no word in Yolngu Matha for hello – but I am to understand that he wants to talk to me. He has signified this; now it is up to me to respond. Time does not press here. I might quite decently delay for hours, but courtesy requires me to respond as surely as if he had phoned me or knocked on my door.

By the time I am free the man might be elsewhere, and it will be up to me to seek him out. I should try to do this today.

I introduce myself to the young man and ask him his name. It is James. He accepts my extended hand. His clasp is soft but he is muscular and well made, and very good-looking. He looks like a triathlete. I ask him whether he wants to talk to me. 'Yes,' he says.

I open the door to Men's Health and stand aside to usher him in, but he hesitates. Gilbert, who interprets for Men's Health, is sitting inside. James does not enter. Instead, Gilbert gets to his feet and abruptly scoots outside and disappears. Only now does James enter and sit down. Now it makes sense: the two men are related, too closely to permit them to speak to each other or to share a room. Gilbert has gracefully made way so we two can speak privately.

'How can I help you, James?'

'Can you give me a checkup?'

I look at him, trying to do this sideways, trying to avoid the direct regard that is a breach of manners, that makes people uncomfortable. Tall and slim, James looks a million dollars, but I ask, 'Are you feeling sick in any way?'

'No, I just want a checkup.'

I look at James' file. He is nineteen. There are no past illnesses of note.

James explains that he has to start work shortly. He has come to see me before starting the new work for his health check.

'What work do you do?'

'I am an apprentice mechanic. I work at the garage. That is my work now, but I want to try for the military. I exercise every day at the gym so they will take me into the Army.'

'Is there anything special you want me to check?'

'Just a checkup, you know ... some tests ...'

What does he want? This is the Men's Clinic – perhaps he has some intimately masculine problem.

'James, do you have a discharge? Does it hurt when you piss?' (What is the right word here? *Urinate* or *micturate* seem absurd; *make water* or *pass water* are mystifying metaphors.)

'No.'

I try another tack: 'Do you have a new sexual partner?'

James looks at me, mystified.

I try again: 'Are you having sex with anyone?'

'No, I don't do that.'

'Not now, or not ever?'

'No. Never.'

An adult virgin is an unexpected discovery, but a career in medicine teaches you that rare conditions do occasionally crop up.

I ask James to take his shirt off. He has an athlete's frame, his shoulders and chest are finely muscled, his belly flat.

Thorough medical examination reveals a young man in prime condition. I tell James this. But he still wants some tests, so I order some, checking for anaemia and, because it's the practice in this clinic to do so, some tests for sexually transmitted diseases.

Afterwards, James responds to my enquiries about his family.

'They are all pretty healthy,' he says. 'My brothers, my Mum and Dad, *my son …*'

Once again it is Kelly who explains. 'Sex is a private, intimate business. He wouldn't be ashamed exactly, just embarrassed to talk about it. He depends upon you to know what he means by a *checkup*, and *some tests*.'

Bombs and stolen babies

Nejesda the nurturer sits next to me on the plane back to the mainland. We stop at Millingimbi, her mother's country. 'Mum can remember Japanese planes flying overhead in 1942. The people didn't know anything about bombs or warplanes.

'There's a big crater in Millingimbi; you can still see it. It was made by a bomb that the Japanese planes dropped there. One man saw the bomb falling out of a plane. He got underneath it to stop it, or to make sure it didn't fall on anyone. He saved everyone … except himself. The planes came again and again, bombing and shooting. The people called out "*Eery*! *Eery*! Witchcraft! Witchcraft!"'

I'm puzzled; Millingimbi doesn't look important in any strategic sense. It's just a pearl in a bracelet of islands in a turquoise sea.

I ask Nejesda the obvious question: 'Why? Why did the planes attack this place?'

She shrugs, gives me one of the half-smiles she uses when she speaks of unaccountable cruelty. She says, 'I don't know why. We don't have oil, nothing here really to bomb …'

Nejesda takes me to see the wreckage of warplanes from that time. There they are, thirty metres from the runway, unmistakeably military – a bit of fuselage here, an engine there, some of a wing over there – massive bits of powerful machines for the taking of life, poignant reminders of the loss of life.

Another question: 'Were any of the Yolngu children stolen?'

'Not many. I don't know why. Perhaps the churches were too

strong up here. But some were taken … my cousin – my third cousin – went to Darwin to give birth. There were complications – she couldn't give birth in Galiwin'ku. In Darwin they told her the baby was dead, stillborn. The hospital people said the baby died from complications. My cousin, she wanted to see the baby. They said, "No, it's not a good time for you to be seeing your baby's body, not when it's passed away."

'She went back to Elcho Island and the family said to the hospital people, "Where's the body? We want the body for burial in our place." But they couldn't get the body. This was in the 1960s.

'Well, that baby wasn't dead. She was a little girl. The hospital people gave her to a Balanda couple. They couldn't have children, you know? They adopted the girl and took her down south to where they lived, to Sydney.

'The girl grew up and she knew she was different. She was black, and she knew she was adopted. She wanted to know her story, her people, her country.

'She was thirty when she met her mother. She found her mother in Galiwin'ku. When she flew in to Elcho, when people heard she was coming, everyone on the island came to the airport. She found her mother by looking and asking everyone she met. She had asked for years. Everything pointed to Arnhem Land, and she asked everywhere until she found people who knew the story of the missing body of a stillborn baby.'

I look at Nejesda's soft face. It is a comfortable face. Nejesda is built for comfort. There is no frown, no animus, just that fractured smile.

'By the time the daughter found her mother, she was married herself, with children back in Sydney. Her life was in Sydney. She saw her Mum and then she went back. They had their lives in separate places.'

Nejesda is quiet for a while. I ask her if she has kids. She smiles, this time a full smile. 'Yes, I've got four that I raise … I'm not their biological mother. There's two brothers, my cousin's boys, aged twelve and fourteen. Their Dad lives in Maningrida. The boys don't like it there. My cousin asked me if I would take them.

'And there's a girl, she's six, my sister's girl. My sister is sick, so I raise her. And my brother, he's in Milingimby. He got depression when he split from his wife. I'm looking after his boy – he's four … my brother's getting a bit better now.

'I can't have children of my own. I've gone from no kids to, like, four!' Nejesda anoints this statement with a full chuckle.

Another silence.

Then, 'There was one other child that was taken. That baby boy was my fourth cousin. His mother had a mental illness. When her baby was born – this was in Gove – they said the same: "Your baby died and we buried it". My cousin was mentally sick. She couldn't fight. Her family said they wanted the body, for burial in its own country, but they couldn't get it. And they couldn't find the burial place in Gove.

'That baby grew up in Tasmania. The Health people told the people who adopted him that his mother didn't want him. He was an adult when he found his mother. He searched and he wouldn't stop until he found his people. He was forty years old when he found his people. He came to his country and they saw each other. But he couldn't stay, either. His life was in Tasmania. That's what he knew, those were the people he knew. Some people said he could sue the government Health people.'

'Is he going to sue?'

Nejesda shrugs.

15. IN A TROOPIE FULL OF DANCERS ON THE WAY TO GARMA

It's Garma time in Nhulunbuy. They say there's a free bus from town to the festival, but no one knows where to catch it or when it leaves. So I wander into town and look for someone who might know.

In Woollies an oldish bloke with a flushed face and not much hair holds a fistful of Cherry Ripe bars. He looks full of purpose. He seems the best prospect: 'Excuse me, mate, do you know where I can catch the bus out to Garma?'

The old bloke looks me up and down and says, 'You want to go to Garma?'

'Yep.'

'Come this way.'

And he leads me into the carpark, to a mud-brown troop carrier with Garma livery on its doors. Inside and outside the troopie are numerous rangy Aboriginal guys and a couple who are comfortably spherical. The Cherry Ripe man hurries the stragglers into the vehicle: 'Let's go, fellers. We don't want to be late.'

They clamber into the back while Mister Cherry Ripe holds the door. He indicates for me to follow. When we have all sat down, there are two in the front, eight of us in the back, and two large bags of Spanish onions and half a dozen packs of Woollies snags underfoot. There are feet and onions everywhere and not much evidence of seat belts – and the atmosphere of hilarity and excitement of a bus full of kids heading off to school camp.

My host extends a hand: 'Ken. And these blokes are dancers from out west of here.'

'Hi Ken. I'm Howard.'

It's a struggle to find the business end of my seat belt. I discover it buried beneath the ample hip of the innermost person on our seat, a woman. After a silent and discreet effort I manage to make myself secure without committing any act of undue familiarity. We lurch and sway around bends and jump potholes and belt along the graded dirt track to Garma. My mind is full of the stories I heard back at the hospital of the head-on that killed two last year on this road.

Meanwhile a sort of negotiation is taking place. The bloke sitting opposite Ken is humbugging him, Ken resisting: 'No, man, definitely not. I haven't got money to give to anyone!'

One round to Ken. There follows a full-length humbug bout, not for money but for something else, something I don't catch. Ken again: 'No mate, no we're not stopping there. Not anywhere. We don't want to be late.'

The man opposite Ken is not giving up. He puts his face in Ken's and raises his voice. A shake of Ken's head. Now the bloke is shouting, now sulking, now slapping the seat next to him, now muttering under his breath – all of this, so far, in a combination of mongrel English and his own language. Then crystal clear, in classic Anglo-Saxon, comes: 'Bullshit! Fucking bullshit! THAT'S. FUCKING. SHIT! ... Fucking. Bloody. Bullshit.' He repeats the phrase a few times, feeling its weight, getting the taste of it, enjoying the ring and the swing of it.

The others in the vehicle, initially mere spectators, have become barrackers, progressively more engaged in the argument. It appears that the shouting man has become their champion, negotiating on behalf of the group. The negotiator is formidable, a wiry bloke of about thirty years with a fierce vitality, mobile features, a repertoire of sounds and expression and a manner seemingly ready at any moment to explode from anger into violence. His squalls of argument are echoed on all sides by an urgent, swelling growl of support.

This seems like a good time to keep a low profile. I keep my head down, my seatbelt snug in my lap and myself to myself, as the troop carrier speeds along the dirt track to Garma.

A glimpse of Ken in my lateral field shows a face set quietly in passivity, neither counter-attacking, nor parrying, nor yet retreating. He is a block, a wall of sandstone, a topographic feature. Not amenable to persuasion. He directs a question to Marcus, our driver: 'How we going for time, Marcus?'

'All right – so long as we don't stop. We're definitely not going to the golf club. We're not stopping.'

Aaah, the golf club – they sell grog there. Now the argument makes sense. Last night the town was awash with alcohol, an unusual event since the Intervention. And we were back to the pre-Intervention days at the hospital, busy all night, suturing and x-raying and repairing the bodies of brothers and sisters and sons and fathers and husbands and wives, all broken by grog rage. I look around at my sullen companions. Were they among the grog-crazed, I wonder?

Ken is handing out the Cherry Ripe chocolate bars. He has seven, one for everyone aboard other than the driver, and me and Ken himself. A quiet falls upon the troopie, people sit back in their seats and abruptly the argument comes to an end.

Seven pairs of jaws chew methodically as Ken tells me about our fellow passengers. 'These people come from a good way west of here. It's their first Garma. They've come to dance. The bloke on your left, he's an elder, a Law Man, very senior in the Law. These fellers opposite, they're his son, his sons-in-law and his nephew; and the lady next to him is Olive, his wife.'

The Law Man chews juicily on his Cherry Ripe and starts to talk. He says something and the others laugh. He speaks again, more laughter. He's looking at me, chewing, saying something; they're all roaring and he puts an arm around me, holds me close and laughs with them. His laughter turns to coughing, also juicy. His face turned towards me, he says something more, laughing and coughing a spray of Cherry Ripe and other fluids in my direction. I look at my trousers, speckled now with dark chocolate. I look up and intercept a volley of liquid chocolate. I haven't eaten one of those wonderful cherry-chocolate bars since I was a kid, but now, as particles of the Law Man's Cherry Ripe cross the threshold of my lips, I recognise that great taste.

Eventually the masticating Law Man finishes his coughing and laughing. Now, with his mouth free again for conversation, he resumes his joke. He clutches me, speaks in language, looks from me to his audience and back, and once again all laugh heartily. Clearly it is a good joke and the joke is me; but I am enjoying it as well. It all feels good-humoured and vastly better than the Great Golf Club Negotiation.

Having thoroughly taken the piss out of me, the joking man decides I am his friend. 'What's your name, brother?'

'Howard.'

That name clearly rings a bell. He pulls his head away and looks searchingly at me.

'No, not John Howard … just Howard.'

'Ohh, that's all right … You can't help that.'

And with that, he introduces me to his fellow dancers, all relatives. Olive, his wife, sensing perhaps that the joking has been hard on me, is keen to put me at my ease. She tells me about the purpose of their trip to Garma. 'We're dancers. We're going to perform our dancing … special dancing, ours only … no one else has this dancing. My husband here, he knows the songs, he is the singer. My brother here,' – she indicates the big roly-poly guy diagonally opposite – 'he plays the didgeridoo. And we all dance.'

Olive is a delightful lady. She explains that her family dances the story of her people and their land and the Law. She shines with pride and satisfaction.

By now brother didgeridoo has finished his Cherry Ripe. He watches hungrily as the skinny fellow next to him rolls a very skinny smoke, lights up and takes a couple of deep drags. Without words, without a look passing between the two men, the smoke changes hands. The larger man cradles the stunted rollie and sucks it down to a glowing speck.

As inconspicuously as I can, I open the window behind me.

Now the big bloke bots a tailor-made and he smokes that one too, drawing hard and quickly, closing my window as he does so, making sure none of that precious smoke escapes.

Someone directs a demand to the driver. Abruptly we stop and all the men take a leak. Olive dismounts with ponderous graceful-ness and crosses the road. All the men turn their backs on her and her husband asks me to do likewise. 'Face away from that side. We gotta show respect.'

Our bladders emptied, we clamber back into the troopie and set off at speed so as not to be late for the dancing.

The hard, wiry man who had demanded earlier to stop off at the golf club ('just for a minute') reaches now into a plastic bag and pulls out lengths of frayed red fabric and passes them around. I watch the Law Man tie a ragged red strip around his head, then the others follow suit.

On an impulse, I extend a hand and ask for a red strip too; then I tie it into a headband and everyone nods and laughs and the Law Man says, 'You dance too, John Howard! You dance with us!'

The troopie takes a bend at speed, we all roll against each other, red onions tumble free, scores of sausages take wing and everyone laughs again.

We pull up at Garma and get out. Just before I part from my friends the dancers, I ask Ken the name of their community. He tells me the name – which I recognise – always mispronounced in the city, a name notorious Australia-wide for the ferocity of the street violence of its gangs at night.

At 4.00 p.m. the great indigenous potentate, celebrated across the nation, takes the mike. It was he who created Garma. He delivers a long, breathy speech hailing the ruling by the High Court of Australia on the Yolngu claim for their traditional waters. Just this past week the court has recognised full native ownership from the high-water mark well out to sea. For the Yolngu it is hugely significant. It is as if the Returned Servicemen's League had applied for recognition of Anzac Day, and after years of waiting, had finally been awarded a legal judgment that expresses the reality.

And now the potentate introduces performers from west of here who will dance and sing the stories of these waters. The faces and limbs of the dancers are dappled with white ochre. Led by six men wielding spears and one rotund woman, all wearing ragged red headbands and red loincloths, they move to the centre of the great space. To the pulsing droning of a didgeridoo played by a round man in red headband and loincloth, they leap into movement. Others join the dance, old men, grey-haired ladies, whip-thin youths and young boys, all watching and following their leaders intently and with great solemnity. Patches of white ochre alternate with black skin, flashing and darkening like ripples catching the sun.

The dance is brief, practically a spasm; it lasts perhaps twenty seconds. Feet stamp, bodies whirl, knees oscillate, bend and straighten and dust rises in an enveloping cloud … and as suddenly as they begin, the dancers stop. They stand, immensely powerful in their stillness, as intensely dramatic in suspension as in movement; and then abruptly they dance again, and once more the trampled earth rises up.

Again and again, the dancers erupt into movement, arrest their dance then resume. Breathless, I watch, one among many hundreds, this enactment of surging tropic tides and cyclonic storms in their abrupt cycles of change. And my wild and stormy friends, the dancers of the western coasts, move and cease, dance and stop, in cycles without end.

16. IN THE KOORI CHILDREN'S COURT

Sitting I

The defendant enters. He is massive, his body broad and deep. Is he truly sixteen years old?

His manner is quiet and watchful. Absent is the swagger, the 'defiance and disrespect' noted by the magistrate on his first attendance here. Somewhere within this precocious bulk and his present docility lies another persona, one that terrorised whole compartments of commuters and car after car full of motorists.

The Clerk calls: 'All stand' then the magistrate enters, a lady in her middle years. She sits, we sit, and she speaks.

'The Children's Court recognises and acknowledges the Wurrundjerri people. We sit today in traditional Wurrundjerri land.' She pauses, then resumes, 'This court has been smoked according to traditional practice.' Another pause as the magistrate allows her words to settle.

Then, 'The Children's Court acknowledges the Wurrundjerri elders – both those present and those past. The court welcomes the following respected persons: Aunty Louisa, Aunty Henrietta and Uncle Willie, who assist the court in today's matters.' The magistrate speaks without legal jargon, but with a measured semi-formality.

This magistrate represents the third generation of her family to officiate in the Children's Court. Outside the court she is known as Lucy. She sits at a large oval table, directly opposite the defendant. If this were a footy oval, the two would be playing on opposite wings. The flanks either side of the magistrate are occupied by Aunties Louisa and Henrietta and by Uncle Willie.

To the right and to the left of the defendant sit a police officer and an older man who is the defendant's lawyer. In the forward and back pockets are two large, well-turned-out indigenous adults who are support persons for the defendant. On either side of them sit an indigenous welfare officer and the defendant's counsellor.

Of eleven people seated at the oval table, seven are indigenous.

Although the magistrate and the defendant are seated at opposite sides of the table they could, if they both wished, reach forward and touch each other. Having heard about the defendant's violent acts on trains and at train stations, I would not relish being touched by him, nor sitting opposite him on a bad day on a train.

And there were some very bad days.

Samuel – that is the name of the defendant – was born prematurely to parents who separated soon after his birth. Samuel's mother's subsequent partners were generally violent towards her and invariably so towards Samuel.

His father has been absent from Samuel's life for most of the sixteen years since then. But when, in recent times, Samuel has sought him out, he has found in his father a person he can recognise.

The police officer reads the statements of the arresting officers of Samuel's two-day rampage six months previously. It takes the officer twenty minutes to read the dry facts. That they are facts is not disputed. Samuel has pleaded guilty to all of the charges.

It was a busy two days.

Day one: closed circuit TV at the outer suburban railway station shows Samuel with mates, drinking. Samuel accosts a young woman, demands her mobile phone, declares it 'a piece of shit' and throws it onto the tracks. The woman flees and Samuel chases her. The footage shows him unable to chase; he sits down and attempts to open a bottle but fails – he is manifestly too drunk.

It is 9.15 a.m.

Samuel boards a train and terrorises passengers all the way from outer Melbourne to an inner suburb. Menacing and threatening, punching the hesitant in the face or head, he steals phones, credit cards, $400 in cash from one passenger, an iPod from another. A thirteen-year-old boy refuses to give up his phone. He pleads with Samuel, says it's his Mum's phone and she'll kill him if he loses it. Samuel hits him in the face with a bottle, fracturing his cheekbone and eye socket, narrowly missing the eye.

He detrains, forces entry to a car, hotwires it and drives into the rear of another car. The car stops, he takes a tyre lever, threatens the other driver, calls her a white dog, forces her from her car and drives it away, leaving her shaken.

Later testimony describes a grandmother who suffers flash-backs and palpitations for months afterward.

On day two there follows a visit to an old people's home where Samuel attempts to smash a reinforced door, then breaks the window of a Honda sedan and drives off in it. He runs another car off the road, threatens to kill the two people in the car – both Sikhs – abusing them racially and robbing them at the point of an eight-inch knife.

He spends the remainder of this day serially stealing, driving, trashing and looting cars. At one stage a police vehicle gives chase, but he eludes it at high speed in heavy suburban traffic.

He is awakened at home the next morning by two police officers who wish to interview him. He admits nothing, makes no comment. They arrest him, leading him past the last of the stolen vehicles, a silent accuser, parked outside in full view.

Samuel was arrested 183 days ago. Since then he has been held on remand. Strikingly, he has expressed a wish not to be released.

Sheltered person that I am, I feel my white middle-class heart beat faster as I listen to the unvarnished facts of one boy's actions on the trains and streets of my city.

Samuel's lawyer, tall, grey, grey-suited, hunched and lined, is Walter Matthau incarnate. Desiccated and academic, he pleads alcohol and cannabis and amphetamines in mitigation of Samuel's actions.

Lucy: 'Alcohol does not excuse this. Drugs do not excuse it. The law does not accept intoxication as a defence.'

Numerous character witnesses, his foster-mother, a Salvation Army youth worker, a cousin, all speak of the Samuel they know, a lovable person, sweet and gentle. The Samuel they know does not take drugs or alcohol.

Samuel's foster-mother has had him since he was twelve. Tall and fair, with her hair in a bun and her pendulous double chin, she looks about sixty-five. She looks like everyone's beloved grandma. She has been fostering kids for thirty years. She starts to speak of the Samuel who helps out at home, that quiet and respectful boy. She cannot reconcile that Samuel with the actions she has just heard described. She stops talking, starts to weep, shaking her head. Her double chin shakes, wet with tears, as she weeps.

She cannot go on.

Samuel's prison welfare worker is an indigenous woman in her forties. She has been around prisons all her working life. Lean, long of limb, she moves with unselfconscious physical gracefulness and poise. With quiet confidence and perfectly pitched clarity, she summarises her observations of the defendant.

She describes Samuel's time in prison, his drying out, his prompt contrition and remorse, his subsequent engagement in Aboriginal cultural studies. She says, 'Samuel has started painting. He paints scenes of himself with his father. Samuel never saw his father much.

'I contacted his great-grandmother – Samuel's father's

grandmother – in Newcastle. She has been a goldmine of information for Samuel about his family, both sides of his family. She has taken Samuel to her heart, she's even come down from Newcastle –twice – to visit him. She's re-connected him with his family. She'd be here today but she's not well enough to travel … Since he met his great-grandmother, Samuel has started to study his Koori heritage, his culture. He wants to become part of the Koori community.'

The magistrate invites the elders to speak. These three are neither sheltered nor white, and they too are shaken.

Aunty Louisa leans forward, her face set, wagging a crooked finger at Samuel, berating him. 'Where's your family from? What's your country? What do you reckon your family thinks of the way you acted? How do you think Koori people like your behaviour?'

Uncle Willie addresses the defendant: 'Samuel, you tell us what were you doing? What were you thinking? You say you want to be part of the Koori community. Let me tell you something – *we don't want you* – we don't want people who behave like you did. We're trying to build ourselves up; people like you break us down. You think for a minute, then tell us: What were you doing? What were you thinking?'

For the first time, Samuel speaks. His voice, a boy's voice, emerges from his mountainous frame. He speaks slowly and quietly. He looks downward, unwilling to meet the elder's glowering gaze. 'I was up early, with friends. We'd been drinking the night before, smoking ganja, taking some pills … About seven of us went down to the station. We had some more to drink …'

Samuel gestures in the direction of the police officer, his voice falls to a whisper: 'You've heard the rest.'

Uncle Willie has more to say. He leans forward, his facial muscles taut, his muscular body straining across the table in Samuel's direction. 'Samuel – smashing someone in the face with a bottle – you could have been on a murder charge! Have you thought about that?'

'Yes.'

Willie's voice has been gathering intensity. Saliva appears at the corners of his mouth as he speaks. His face creases as he hammers his words home: 'When you run around making the streets and the roads and the trains unsafe for ordinary people, when you terrify people, when you steal and trash, you *are* trash. You make us ashamed.'

Now Willie is thundering. 'What we Kooris are filthiest about is racism! Those young blokes from India, they come here to study, their parents work and save and send them here to learn, and what sort of impression do you give them of our country? What will they say back home in India about Kooris?'

Uncle Willie has finished speaking. For a long moment he holds Samuel's gaze in an unremitting glare. The court is rigid with the moment, with the transaction between an elder and a boy. It feels like a critical encounter, an initiation.

Now Aunty Henrietta speaks: 'Samuel, how long have you been on remand?'

'Six months, miss.'

'And you don't want to come out?'

'No, miss.'

'Why not?'

'I'm scared I'll go backwards, Miss ...'

'Well, I agree with you, Samuel. You're not ready to go out. And when you do, you get yourself a new set of friends. Those friends of yours – at the station, on the train – they're not your friends. The drugs, the grog, they're no good to you, they're no good for us Kooris. Tell me – do any of your relatives want to know you?'

Faces look up and crane backwards at a minor disturbance in the rear of the court. The rear door is held open for a longish minute, but no one enters or leaves. Finally, a baby's pusher noses into the body of the court with a young couple in close attendance.

They are both thin. The man is fair, the woman pale. The man wears a suit to which his long, lean body seems a stranger. He swims in it.

The man – in reality he appears more a boy than a man – leans forward and delicately, deliberately unbuckles and hoists a very small baby into the arms of the young woman. She sits down and holds the baby to her breast. I look up and catch the expression on the face of the defendant; he is beaming.

The court is altered. Everyone (except Walter Matthau) seems to be smiling. Alive to this, the magistrate asks, 'Samuel, do you have any relatives here to support you?'

'Yes, your Honour,' – he indicates the couple and their baby – 'my cousin, your Honour.'

'You seem to have a lot of support in this court, Samuel. Despite everything, these people still have faith in you. You would not want to disappoint them.'

'No, your honour.'

'I am going to adjourn this hearing, Samuel. The court will wait a few months more before I decide – and it will be my decision alone, not the elders', not the Police – whether you have a long sentence or some other judgement. I want some more time to think about your future, and you need to think as well; you need to think about how you want to spend the rest of your life. Where you want to spend it.

'Meanwhile I am going to give you certain guidelines and conditions; and I advise you seriously to observe them between now and next time you come here.'

Between sittings

I thought Uncle Willie looked familiar; I was right. Twenty years ago, he was one of the fittest men in the country and one of the most vilified. In popular estimation, he held the highest judicial office in the land as a senior referee in football. In his jurisdiction, he held matters weightier to barrackers than mere life and death. On the field he was treated with prudent respect. From beyond the boundary he was called a black maggot. It is easy to see in today's lean, muscular man the athlete of yesterday.

I have a question for Willie: 'What does it mean that the court-room has been smoked?'

'Smoking is the way we purify something. It can be a penance, a peacemaking with the spirits of a place. After a death, we smoke the room where the dead person lay. In the court here, we smoke it to make it clean, to make a new start.'

⊚⊚⊚

Some five decades ago the court's present judicial officer was also known to me as a fair-haired teenage girl called Lucy. She explains the singular style and structure of the court to me: 'Everything – the welcome to country, the presence and participation of the elders, the standing given to non-judicial indigenous persons – everything is geared to making this anything but a white persons' court.

'We find that the advice and exhortations of the respected persons carry real weight. We often find that the elders are more severe on an offender than the magistrate.

'A crucial distinction of this court is prior acquaintance or connection. Invariably one of the respected persons knows or is related to someone involved in the case. This would disqualify an official in other courts; here it is unavoidable and actually indispensable. When an elder person speaks to an offender, the fact of connection creates gravitas. Otherwise we would be as irrelevant as any other centre of white authority.

'Like all children's courts, we try to create a second – or third, or fourth – chance for our kids. We are not always successful. Look at this poem. It was written by an indigenous child offender in another state.'

I won't be here long
I came here first
After my terrible thirst.
I spilled some blood –
Mine and another's mixing in mud.
I came here, my temper had burst
And they gave me a chance
To do my best – after my worst,
But my life is a dance.
I got my chance wrong.
This is the song
The song of my grog,
The song of my bong.
I won't be here long.

'This was found in a holding cell. The offender was only seventeen. He was found hanging in his cell, dead.'

Sitting II

The magistrate looks across the oval table to the defendant. 'We are here today, Samuel, to resume your case.'

Lucy consults her notes and when she speaks her tone is friendly. She starts by congratulating him on his good record since his last appearance. She is pleased that the court has heard no further reports of misbehaviour. She speaks of his good response to counselling. She notes that he has visited his mother and his siblings on day leave, and on overnight leave. She is pleased to hear that he is helping Mum with the new baby, and that the other kids at home look up to him and model themselves on him.

Lucy notes that Samuel has been going out to TAFE for schooling and doing his homework. At this, she stops speaking and looks hard at him. She says, 'That's very, very important, Samuel, very pleasing.'

And in his regular absences from custody, he has not absconded.

Lucy calls for reports from the oval table. Samuel's counsellor reports on Samuel's visits to his father. His father is in jail, his principal place of residence over most of Samuel's years. Samuel and his father have the same story: violent childhood, split and centrifugal nuclear families, early and constant alcohol abuse, drug abuse, school failure, absenteeism and criminality. Same story, different chapters. Both are looking to change their scripts.

The counsellor speaks of Samuel's painting. He is taking lessons. His paintings are of himself, his father and the dreaming motif that his great-grandmother taught him. He is immersing himself in Koori cultural studies. He seizes the reading material that his counsellor brings him from the community's library. He says he wants to become a part of the Koori community.

Samuel's lawyer reports that Samuel's blood and urine tests for drugs and alcohol have remained negative.

Samuel's TAFE report is read out. It refers favourably to attendance, completion of homework, enthusiastic involvement in the art elective and to his commencement of trade studies.

'What trade would you like to follow, Samuel?' asks the magistrate.

'I'm doing hairdressing, your Honour. I want to have my own hairdressing business.'

For the first time I notice Samuel's hair. Cut short and styled in tight curls, thoroughly anointed with 'product', it is the head of a young god. Samuel holds that head modestly bowed as the Aunties banter with him: 'We'll come to you for a cut and some colour when you start up your salon, Samuel.'

The magistrate invites the elders to speak to Samuel.

Aunty Louisa: 'You're doing well, son. Keep it up; don't go backward. You're discovering something all of us Kooris get to know – *you can't change the past, but you can make the future different.*'

Aunty Henrietta: 'I saw in your report how you read the victims' statements and you were ashamed … as you should be!

And how you wrote to the boy you hit with the bottle and to the Indian students, that you were sorry and you wanted to meet them face to face.'

'Yes, miss.'

'That's a start. That's a good start, Samuel.'

On this occasion Uncle Willie's body speaks a different language. Leaning back in his chair, speaking softly, Willie might be talking with a friend at their club. An intimacy has been born between the two. 'When you were here last time, I said the Koori community would not want you the way you were. Well, it looks to me like you're different now. The way you're going, you could make a contribution to the community. You're going well.

'One more thing: you heard the magistrate say how the court has been smoked in the way of our tradition. I want you to think about that, what it means. Take it to heart, son.'

Everyone has spoken. The courtroom sits quietly as the magistrate gathers her papers together. At the back of the court a baby sucks audibly on its dummy. The magistrate speaks to Samuel: 'This court has heard only good of you in the months since you were taken into custody. It is clear that everyone here is pleased and impressed with how you've turned your life around.

'You have been in custody now for nine months. That is a large piece out of a young life. The harm you did was very great. Imprisonment for twice that period would not be too long. I have decided not to confine you those extra nine months ...' – here the magistrate pauses. 'Instead, you will be on probation. At the end of today's hearing, you will be released under the supervision of a probation officer. There will be very strict conditions imposed upon you during that period.

'You will attend this court once more, nine months from now. If in that time you have not re-offended, you will leave the court a free person. I should say – a free man.

'We – the elders and I, your counsellor, your support people, your family – we do not want to see you here before then.'

Samuel looks up. He turns to his lawyer. He appears perplexed. A whispered conversation, then Walter Mathau says, 'Samuel has a question, Your Worship.'

'What is it, Samuel?'

'When I'm on probation, will I still not be allowed to go on trains?'

'No, that restriction will not continue … Do you mind telling the court, why is that important to you?'

'Your Honour, I want to be able to take Mum to the city for the sales.'

17. OMERTÀ

I cannot swear to the truth of everything that follows here. I write here of some things that I do not see with my own eyes. I hear about them from others. And some of my informants are saying what they have heard from others. Almost all of this is hearsay. Few victims come forward, no eyewitness supports these reports.

I write here about things that nobody sees but everyone claims to know.

◎◎◎

In every community I visit, doctors affirm the prevalence of sexual abuse of children.

In the whitefella community where I have worked for thirty years, a survey of patients I referred for psychological counselling found that *fifty per cent* had a buried past of sexual abuse. And of course, at the time of referral this GP had no idea: these patients were simply sleepless or anxious or depressed or abusing alcohol or dependant on dope or cutting themselves or hurting their wives ...

In Aboriginal communities female nurses collect data that shows beyond dispute the high incidence of sexually transmitted disease in children. So we do know – *by inference* – that sexual abuse of children is common.

Government reports and enquiries make it official. The

cloyingly named 'Little Children are Sacred' report triggers a government reaction and over-reaction.

Here and there, older women, grandmothers and great-grandmothers, fearless by now of consequences, tell the story: children are being abused sexually. It happened to them when they were small, it happened to their own boys and girls, now they see their grandchildren going through it.

One toddler shows what she has suffered or seen, what she has anyway learned. She lies down, removes her underwear and invites a small boy, a few years her senior – *'You wanna fuck me?'*

Yet in my clinical work in forty to fifty separate locum terms, I do not discover a single case. Is it on account of my being a 'here today, flying out tomorrow' doctor that no one speaks to me?

Even my colleagues – 'stay-here' doctors, trusted, adopted by the local clan, honoured with a skin name – even these learn by hearsay; but only in cases of the greatest extremity does a family come forward and complain.

☺☺☺

Communities have local political leaders as well as traditional elders, both exercising real power and protecting and extending it by various means.

I visit one semi-dry community where a powerful person operates. Recognised by whitefella governments as a leader, some in his community claim he is nevertheless not a traditional head. He lacks the lineage, he lacks the Law. As a result there are some who feel their rightful position has been usurped. The man has rivals and foes.

This man is a permitted drinker while many in his community are not. He has access to large official funds and he has a large, powerful personality. Opponents are cowed. Good governance goes out the window as the leader goes out the door, taking with him funds for 'communal wellbeing'. He spends those funds on grog, feeds it to strategic allies, cronies, satellites, who fall, grateful and helpless in that incoming tide.

When, later, those people want more grog, they fall into line with the powerful man and do his bidding. Soon he is controlling his community by means of his permitted alcohol.

The misappropriated funds are substantial, the wrongdoing quietly but broadly notorious. Amazingly, government does not know. Some people in government, powerful people, know that it is better not to know. Better for them, their career, their budget, their power.

When I hear these whispers I wonder whether I am hearing envy speaking. But my informant does not come from this remote community. He is not indigenous. Surely he has nothing to fear. But, I reason, perhaps *his* informant is lying. I put the whispers aside.

The days pass. Daily, non-permit persons weave and flow into the clinic, many of them the worse for drink. To this there are eye-witnesses – the nurse and the doctor. Who gives the grog to these people?

More whispers. Non-indigenous whisperers, all non-eyewitnesses, all speak in whispers to protect their informants.

From what? From whom?

Every one of the potentates has opponents, rivals, clan enemies, but even among the enemies no one steps forward. No one breaks the silence.

◎◎◎

In Sardinia there is an organisation called the *Camorra*. The *Camorra* manages the flow of information within its communities by bribery, threats, murder, kidnappings and ties of kin. Disputes and grievances are settled within the organisation. They do not call the police.

The code of secrecy of the *Camorristi* is called *Omertà*.

◎◎◎

I wonder why silence is pervasive in Aboriginal communities. This is not Sardinia; but the coercive silence is just like *Omertà*. Why do victims and political foes not come forward? What, or whom, might they fear?

Non-indigenous informants who speak to me of sexual violence and of corrupt leaders explain the silence of others in a whisper: 'Sure, some are frightened. A traditional leader has magical powers, frightening powers of harm.

'In a case of child abuse, can you imagine a small girl speaking up against someone older and bigger? Most often it's a relative. Sometimes an elder.'

'But,' I ask, 'even people who are beyond fear – grandmothers, older women – why do so few speak up?'

'Shame! The shame of having been raped. The shame of speaking of things like that in front of an outsider, especially a male. And when a respected leader is corrupt, there's the community's feeling of shame about that. The pain of speaking up, that shame would be worse than the experience of being bullied or ripped off by their head person.'

◎◎◎

Within the Melbourne Jewish community, there exists a small group of devout individuals who live a rigorously traditional life, closed off from the secular world. The group observes a very strict code of purity and sanctity. Their houses do not have TV, their children attend gender-segregated schools within that community, all dress with a degree of modesty paradoxically comparable to that of strict Muslims. This is not a wealthy group. Many are poor.

I refer to the group as a sect because it is just that, *cut off*, dissected away from the world of secular Jews and other orthodox groups, by clear choice. In indigenous terms, sect members live in a town camp within and separate from the rest of Melbourne Jewry. They are proud and intensely private.

When, in 2008, reports appeared on the front page of the mainstream Melbourne broadsheet of a sexual scandal within the sect, the trauma was intense. Allegations were made that a venerated senior educator within the community had sexually molested a number of students of the same gender. The students were traumatised, their parents stricken, the entire group shaken.

The perpetrator was allowed to leave the community unscathed, reportedly in possession of scarce community funds. The departure of the miscreant ahead of police action was actively aided by members of the community.

The motivation for the protection of the abuser appeared to lie in the shame felt by the community. It seems that the publicity hurts even more than the abuse itself.

Everything I write here about this scandal exists already in the public domain. Yet I tremble physically as I write this. I, knowing no one in that sect personally, I whose life is lived entirely separately, feel a physical reaction to speaking out.

The thing about *Omertà*, the powerful thing, is its communal roots, its networks of safety and harm.

PART FOUR

HOPE

The day is short, the work is great ... the Master is
pressing ... It is not incumbent upon you to complete
the task, but neither are you free to absolve yourself of it.

(Ethics of the Fathers 2:15-16, Babylonian Talmud)

18. THE PAINTER OF YIRRKALA

The painter sits on the floor, his paints arrayed at his feet, his painting between his knees. The pigments are brilliant – vivid greens, blazing reds and orange, luminous blues and turquoise, stark black, a shining white – all lying at his feet in their uncapped tubes, a spectrum of energy in potential, awaiting translation into a composed work on paper.

Respectfully, I stand a little behind and to the side of the painter, hoping not to let my watching presence disturb his flow. I have seen Aboriginal painters at their work before, at Desart in Alice, and at Warlayirti Arts in Balgo. Like this artist, they work seated on the floor, bent forward over their work, their brushes and paints scattered around their feet. But this painter is different; he and I have a relationship, as patient and doctor.

My patient flew to this hospital a couple of days ago, unable to breathe properly. At present, he is a nine-fingered painter: an electronic probe sits like a thimble over the tip of his left fifth finger, monitoring the oxygen saturation of his blood. He has hypoxia, a condition that creates an anxious feeling and agitation. His breathing is a labour, born of the joint efforts of his heaving diaphragm and the straining muscles in his chest. Even the muscles of his neck have been recruited to the pursuit of breath. The noises of this labour are rhythmic and relentless: a fast gasping as he sucks air in, a rattling and growling as he squeezes the dead air out. In, out, in, out. I stand, quietly appalled, fighting down my own agitation.

But my patient the painter paints on imperturbably.

The 'canvas' is small, really just a sheet of A4 torn from a book of art paper. A margin of black has been painted onto the paper. I stand and watch as the artist transforms the empty expanse of white into something that lives. Unhurried, unhesitating, unerring, he dips into blobs of pigment expressed from the tubes then transfers the paint, dot by blazing dot, onto the page.

Within moments the page is alive.

I move on, drawn by the more urgent need of even sicker patients, away from this scene of creation and birth.

When I return only twenty minutes later, the painting is complete. From margin to black margin the paper is covered entirely with brilliant dots.

The patient's mother lifts her son and offers the breast. He is three years of age.

19. BIDYADANGA, PETAKH TIKVAH

In 1886, my grandfather was born in Petakh Tikvah, a small settlement across the sand dunes from Jaffa, in Turkish Palestine.

Tel Aviv did not yet exist and the desert had not bloomed. Someone, some dreamy optimist, was inspired to give the windblown settlement that name. It means 'Gateway of Hope'.

One hundred and ten years after my grandfather left his birthplace, I find myself in another dry and sandy place on a coast, another gateway of hope. It is in the Kimberley, in the northwestern corner of Australia, a couple of hundred kilometres south of Broome. Its name is Bidyadanga. It is the largest Aboriginal community in Western Australia.

They say the population of Bidyadanga is nine hundred souls. A problematic statistic: how do the census takers count souls? I accept that there are nine hundred people alive and walking around. Many, many more lie in small anonymous graves. Each grave is marked by a small wooden cross, placed there by the mission when a young child in their care passed away. There are no names. These children were stolen. (Not the fault of the mission, as far as I can see. They received and cared for the children; they never stole them.)

Where are the souls of the stolen children, I wonder. For indigenous people, such questions are emphatically not idle. Recently some (not all) European museums returned to Aboriginal hands human 'specimens' that were taken from their country a century or more ago. A museum is an institution with pretensions to scientific purpose and records. Thus it was possible to return many of the remains precisely to their places of origin. The return to the custodians of country was marked by the most passionate oratory I have ever heard for persons long nameless, long dead.

Serious ceremony followed as tribal remains were accorded their fitting rites. All this to allow the spirit to find rest. With return comes recovery of the indefeasible unity between Aboriginal body and ancestral land. That unity recognises no distinction between fauna and flora and land and Law.

The small nameless graves of Bidyadanga lie surrounded by long grass. The traveller has no intuition of a burial ground and skirts these long grasses unaware. The trade winds sough, the grasses wave, the souls of these lost children continue the endless wait for their own country …

◎◎◎

My wife and I drive the 200 kilometres from Broome to Bidgy with the regular doctor, Dr Larni, a young woman who gives us cheerless and cheerful news: 'The town is supposed to be dry. There's a community statute that prohibits the sale and importation of alcohol here. But people fill up their car boot elsewhere and bring the grog into town …' We discover it is pretty much soaked with grog; it is possibly Australia's foremost diabetes training ground (fifty per cent incidence), and it has an astonishing rate of kidney disease requiring dialysis. And few of the people have real work.

Yet for all its sorrowful past and its patchy present, Bidyadanga of today is a place of hope.

Dr Larni continues: 'About half the people drink and about half go to church. There are two churches here and they're both going strong. One's been here forever – that's the Catholic Church, and the other is newer – they're the Assemblies of God. The Catholics have a crackerjack young minister from the Philippines.'

Would I normally be encouraged by a fifty-fifty ratio between drinkers and non-drinkers? Probably not. Perhaps I have just been infected with the doctor's enthusiasm. This young lady is probably half my age. She is completing her Fellowships in General Practice and in Rural and Remote Medicine; she has already done a Diploma in Child Health, and is about to enrol in the Master of Public Health program.

Larni comes from down south. She's been here for a year-and-a-half and has no plans to move on. Her time in Bidgy has coincided with a great increase in funding and resources for the clinic; they're recruiting and retaining lots of Aboriginal health workers, and the local health workforce is skilful and motivated. And stable.

Unspoken but encouraging to me is the fact of Larni's continuity. People are getting to know and trust her. Larni is typical of her generation of remote doctors. Patients who bewail the passing of the multi-skilled, dedicated country doctor should look at the outback. Happily, it is indigenous people who are the beneficiaries of these gifts.

We drive into town. The Olympic-size swimming pool gleams, brilliant in the afternoon sun. More good news: when a town has a swimming pool, ear infections are halved. Apparently it's all a matter of snot management. Fewer ear infections, better hearing, better learning – that's the pattern. But the best news about the Bidgy pool is the local rule: schoolchildren may only swim if they have been to school that day.

Next morning I miss the bus. Who would guess there'd be a bus in a town of this size? It is the school bus. This, I learn, is a walking bus. The Principal and all the teachers meet early in the morning at the school, then walk together and pick up all the children from their homes. They walk from house to house, waiting for the kids to come out. Would-be truants cannot resist the fun or the peer pressure or the personal pull of the teachers. They all come out and they all *walk* to school.

The school itself has a stable and able staff, young and enthusiastic. School attendance is high. At work I meet Possum Stephens, a national treasure. His tremendous prestige and influence are not confined to this community. And Possum is not alone; there appears to be a culturally intact generation of elders here. That endows a community with structure, with a known history, with people who carry and teach Law. The young prosper; pride grows.

◎◎◎

My wife and I are looking for the new Arts Centre, perhaps to buy something. We have heard the remarkable story of the very recent birth of an entire new school of painting, principally among the old people here. But we are disappointed; with the astonishing success of the painters, all sales take place in the Short Street Gallery in Broome.

The new art movement was largely brought into being under the stimulus of a local teenager who encouraged the old people to make a return to the desert country of their childhood, after initially forcible and now unnecessarily prolonged separation. The old people did return and, culturally refreshed and inspired, began painting. Their young 'leader', now nineteen, is a finalist in 2008's Telstra Indigenous Art Awards. What will this mean for Bidyadanga's future? Past experience shows that leading artists neither bring communal betterment, nor enjoy better personal health. But the art movement in Bidyadanga is unusual. It emerges from an alliance between elders and the young. Perhaps Bidgy can break the mould.

My boss in the Kimberley is a veteran. She tells me that Bidyadanga genuinely appears to have a negligible incidence of child sexual abuse. 'It was difficult for me to believe what I heard. But I heard it from all quarters, from doctors, from nurses, health workers, social workers, sexual health workers. I heard it and I keep hearing it. Now I believe it. And we have the facts and figures that show our little children are healthier today than a few years ago.'

⊚⊚⊚

Reviewing all these hopeful portents, some six months after that short visit to Bidyadanga, my high hopes read like diagnostic features in a personality profile. They might tell a reader more about the frame of mind of this optimist than about the world he sees.

However, the good news trickles in. It comes from all points. The flow carries with it an endless load of odd facts and figures. I begin to gather and retain statistics of good news like the terminal moraine of a glacier.

In Halls Creek, students now receive a nutritious breakfast and lunch every day. School attendance has doubled as a result. Critics argue that this practice disempowers parents. Meanwhile, the kids learn better with a full tummy and their nutrition can only improve.

A pilot research study has been carried out in a remote school. In this experiment, every child was given two pieces of fruit a day. After only six months, antibiotic prescriptions and absenteeism were halved, hearing testing results were better, all markers of health showed improvement. Daily cost per student of this breakthrough intervention is less than a dollar.

Fitzroy Crossing has an Aboriginal-owned pub, long famous for its colossal per capita sales. This pub killed more Aboriginal people than any other. Belatedly, the community clipped the pub's wings: the sale of full-strength beer was restricted and immediately the rate of arrest and injury from violence plummeted.

The hospital's casualty department is quiet at night. With the slowing inflow of grog in the Territory, alcohol-related hospital attendance has fallen by fifty per cent in some places, eighty per cent in others.

141

Since the Federal Government's Intervention, the community of my Garma dancers has received twenty-six new houses. More are being built.

Thursday Island has a population of only 3700 people, served by five alcohol outlets. The list of houses of worship on the island is much longer. It includes the Quetta Anglican Memorial Church, the Sacred Heart Catholic Church, the Uniting Church, the Seventh Day Adventist Church, the Assembly of God, the Full Gospel Church, the Church of Torres Strait, the Church of Jesus Christ of Latter Day Saints and the Independent Church of Torres Strait and Kaiwalagal. In addition there is an impressive Baha'i establishment fronting the main street.

I meet a keen church musician and chorister seconded to Ngurupai; he reckons this list is incomplete. He assures me he knows of numerous additional congregations on Thursday Island.

What, if anything, does all this signify?

During a visit of seventeen days and nights to Ngurupai, the second most populous island in the Torres Strait, I do not encounter a single drunk person. I walk the unlit streets at night and I hear no cries, no crazed shrieks of laughter, none of the sounds of the hooning youth that pollute the nights elsewhere.

Each morning I run the roads and tracks of the island and count abandoned wrecked vehicles. In the course of my long runs I find only seven wrecks on an island of 654 persons.

Seven car hulks, zero drunks, in seventeen days in an Aussie country village. It's un-Australian.

☉☉☉

More ambiguous, because untested, are the radical plans of the indigenous leadership in Cape York country. These ambitious plans are underwritten by very serious whitefella philanthropy. They include overturning welfare; *removal* – by consent – of children for serious schooling, away from abuse in their troubled communities;

real job training with guaranteed real employment to follow – these are initiatives of breathtaking audacity.

Most radically, the Cape York leaders argue explicitly for individual bank savings, personal bank loans and mortgages, and private home ownership. A generation of Aboriginal capitalists will arise.

To an outsider these policies seem to confront and affront ancient cultural norms. In particular, they threaten violence to traditions of collective action and communal ownership. Only an indigenous leader could propose them. Will they speed an end to grog welfare or an end to culture?

Or both?

In all the confusion and contradiction of signs, in all the pain and squalor, when light separates itself from heat and sparks are seen from so many quarters, why should one not hope?

20. POSSUM STEPHENS

Bidyadanga sits on an endless beach with its back to the desert. Its peoples are various; four separate tribes came in from a nomadic life in the desert in a modern exodus that is one of the great untold sagas of this continent. But the fifth tribe of Bidyadanga was always coastal. These saltwater people have been here forever.

Bidyadanga's desert peoples arrived here in a series of immigrations in the third quarter of the twentieth century. Until the fifties and sixties these were desert nomads; some had never seen white men, others had seen them at a distance and kept them there. But family by family, clan by clan, straggling from their places of dune and singing winds they yielded to drought and famine or to the government people who rounded them up and 'brought them in'.

From a place where time was measured by sun, by phases of the moon and by the seasonal migrations of game, they entered a place of clocks, and schools, and churches and doctors.

There are people still alive in Bidyadanga who were born in the desert and who carry memory and story of that life of austere riches.

Led by their teenage grandson, a cluster of the very oldest of these desert people of Bidyadanga returned recently to their country. Their joy on finding intact, buried under sands and time, a remembered desert spring, a *jila*, was recorded on videotape. The footage captures the intensity of this reunion with that site of immense spiritual meaning. These ancients were once again whole. The *jila*, a secret place of permanent water in the desert, has sustained and defined the people, always, beyond all memory, beyond memories of memory, ever beyond time, to the Dreaming that never ends.

☉☉☉

Possum Stephens is a vivacious man. When I meet him in Bidyadanga, his bony face lights up the room. He is, he informs me, 'the heldest in the Law in this country'. Tall and lean, with an ancient hearing aid in one ear, hard of seeing as well, he speaks slowly, in near-circular sentences that make their way slowly across the rough terrain of English.

He is clearly an old man. Officially, his year of birth is 1934. That was the recording official's best guess. Possum says he is 'seventy-four, might be eighty-four, could be ninety-four.' The middle estimate seems about right to me – for what it's worth.

And in Possum's scale of chronology a decade is not worth much, a breath in the winds of timeless time.

I wonder whether Possum is a member of one of the four clans that came in from the desert and settled in this coastal settlement last century. They came, these reclusive nomads, drawn slowly by long drought to the government ration station. Others 'came in' to work on the large cattle station here, yet others were stolen and ended up here in the care of the church.

I ask Stephens, 'Are you a desert man?'

Possum bends and turns his aided ear towards me. It is a movement not of age or of decrepitude but of physical grace. There's that smile again, bathing me. Shining he says, 'No, I'm saltwater man, freshwater man. This my country, this one here. This my place, all this, this Frazier Downs country, used to be ration station … all my country.'

Possum tells me about his people's successful claim for these ancestral lands: 'Big lawyers, three lawyers, from Melbourne, from Sydney, I take them everywhere, I show them my country ...' Possum led the three through his country, from its northern extreme to its southernmost edge, and westward to its inland margin. His narrative makes clear that as the senior traditional owner, he, Possum, was the defining witness to his people's claim. He convinced the court, carried the day for his people, and he is proud of that.

He has a whitefella book that records the facts: 'It's all in the book, that book at my place, all this country, all Law. You can come and look at that book, Doctor.'

Possum tells me he does not read or write. He can sign his name, and he demonstrates that skill, forming letters that are large, round and spiky, ciphers in an uncracked code. Possum never went to school. He was given the Law by his father and his father's father, by uncles, by older brothers-in-law, as they walked and criss-crossed their lands; that was his schooling. That he cannot read the writing in his own book, the lawyers' book of his own country, weighs upon Possum not at all. He knows the Law, he holds the Law. That is everything. The book attests to the truth, but the book is a mere artefact of that truth, good for people who read, good for people who do not hold the Law.

As I sit and listen to this slow-speaking old man, this elder, this man at once gaunt and radiant, time begins to fall away. Possum tells me how he passes on the Law – 'my big Law, ceremony Law' – to his following generations. 'I take 'em, I show 'em: "Don't go there – that secret ground; go there. This one here, this meeting ground ..."'

Time is the medium of all my living reality. But as Possum's account of himself and his land and his Law spirals and tumbles unevenly from him, I begin to shed this chrysalis of my own time and to enter into Possum's world.

In white man time, the government men came and fed the

blacks at the ration station; then the Church came, built the mission and took over from the government; then the mission went away and the government came again.

In Possum's abiding reality, governments come and will also pass. *The lone and level sands stretch far away* ... Clearly I am in thrall of my guest who is, in deeper truth, my host.

Afterwards I scrutinise my reactions: have I romantically imagined or wishfully thought a man after my own dreaming? How much is real? Irreducibly real is a man of great charm and winning gesture, a courtly man of rare self-possession. Possum knows who he is, what he is, what is his, where he belongs.

If I had met a hereditary aristocrat on his estates in Europe, would I feel this deep impression, I wonder? Those estates would be smaller, that lineage shallower, the European culture an infant in comparison. This is Possum Stephens, no less; this man is the eldest in the Law in his country.

Beyond the personage, I enquire about the person who is Possum: 'Do you have children?'

He ponders, looking at me as if it is a trick question. He looks away. At length he says, 'I had seven ... I've got four girls.'

I am not heartless enough to address the deficit. I ask about the girls. They are dispersed around the state: one in Perth, two others are in the Kimberley, one of them here in Bidyadanga.

A pause. 'Did you ever work with cattle?' This lights him up and sets him going. I hear him enumerate the stations where he worked; I hear of his working life in the saddle, and he refers without rancour to the wages: 'They pay me flour and tea, you know, flour, sugar, tobacco. I like that work, horses, cattle. The stations, all stations, they want me to work for them.'

Then Possum reverts to his children. 'My boy, he worked cattle too ... with me ... He died, his horse crashed.' Possum relates the story of the horrific two-horse collision that took his boy; how he, Possum, watched his son, riding at the gallop, taken out by another horseman who, unsighted, galloped into his path from an angle. The horsemen were thrown. One horse landed on Possum's son and broke his neck.

Outside the window little kids are riding their tiny bikes. They ride with all the flair and abandon of cattlemen at a rodeo, but these kids ride on footpaths and wear helmets.

◎◎◎

Mollie is another old person, like Possum, blind and frail. She has come today to have her prescriptions renewed.

Mollie comes from desert country. She has lived here in Bidyadanga now for sixty years, since her early teens. While the nurses restock her dosette box, she tells me about her life here. She too had many children: 'I've got daughters, five, four now … I had three boys. They're not here now. One in Kununurra, one in Halls Creek.'

I am curious about the ones not accounted for but I cannot bring myself to push Mollie where tired memory holds ancient pain at a distance.

'Do you have anyone at home to help you, Mollie?'

'I don't need much help … one daughter with me. Two more not far. Some of them died. Two boys left, one at Argyle mine.

'My husband not alive now. Long time now. In the night I wake up, every night I look for my husband. I don't find him. Then I cry.'

21. A VIOLENT FATHER

I have always enjoyed visiting Ballarat, the location of the beginning of my family's history in this country. In 2008, I visited Ballarat and encountered the future.

At the Base Hospital they boast about the maternal health of indigenous mothers; their birth weights are *better* than the mainstream. They tell me that employment stands at eighty per cent among indigenous adults, and school attendance averages eighty per cent as well.

I visit the Aboriginal Cooperative (the Co-op). The CEO is a brown-skinned lady. She looks different from the other indigenous persons at the Co-op. She is a realist and a fiscal disciplinarian. She regards most politicians and bureaucrats as fools. And she doesn't suffer fools.

I ask her whether the Wutherong are her people. 'No. I'm a Maori.'

She sends me to the highly successful antenatal clinic which will be in action this morning. I am shown into a large airy room that looks like a kindergarten. In fact the room doubles as a crèche; but this morning is Young Mums' morning.

I can't see any nurses or patients, only small children and babies and mothers. And a couple of women without kids, who might be anything.

A young woman wanders in, carrying a newborn baby. The baby is very new. So is the mum: she looks about sixteen. Everyone gathers around, embracing mum, congratulating her, admiring baby, celebrating the new family. Kids crane, toddlers clamber onto chairs to see, to touch the baby.

I look hard at the mother. Too thin, fair, pale, uncertain, she looks very much the new mother, a child herself, vulnerable.

One of the unattached women pulls up a chair for her and fetches another for herself. Other mothers pick up the baby, serial cuddles follow. The seated woman asks questions, listens as the girl answers, nods, rests a hand on her slender shoulder. The woman is twice the girl's age, just about old enough to be her mother. They talk for some time, their conversation punctuated by the arrival of latecomers who flock and kiss and congratulate, then peel off to see the baby.

The baby cries. Experienced hands hold her against large chests to soothe her to sleep. Briefly the baby subsides, then squalls again. They bring baby to the young mum. As she takes the baby I see her stiffen. She unbuttons her shirt and offers the breast. Quiet. Then the baby cries again. The older woman says something, mum nods and allows the older woman to adjust the baby's position. Baby sucks, mum relaxes and the large room breathes out.

◎◎◎

There are wide sliding doors that open onto a large sunny deck. Here bigger kids, three and four and five years old, play and compete for ride-on toys. The sunshine wins me and I turn my back on the antenatal clinic where no one seems to be pregnant, and go outside.

I find a seat and spend some time absorbing photons and doing not much else. I am not the only adult here. One of the bigger kids is playing with a man who could be her dad. They have a soccer ball and not much room. The girl wants to play 'football'.

Under his right arm the man holds a baby. With his left arm the man plays football the way his daughter demands. She stands two metres distant and tells him to roll the ball to her. He does so. She rolls it back. Backwards and forwards the ball rolls in a lulling rhythm.

For quite some time the girl is highly satisfied. Eventually, worn out by these exertions, she puts down the ball, picks up a book and gives it to dad to read.

About this time the underarm baby starts to cry and dad stops reading, sniffs the nappy and goes inside for a nappy bag. He emerges with a round lady who changes the soiled nappy while the story resumes. The baby suckles on a bottle as I offer the lady my seat and go back inside.

Inside the room, the crowd has thickened. More mums, more toddlers, more babies. Some of the mothers have only a first baby, others have more. They chat and cuddle and swap babies and they breastfeed.

I notice a handful of young women with big bellies. The ante-natals have started to arrive. And the two unattached women move from one to another, talking, listening, watching. No one addresses these two as 'Nurse'. They are just women among other women, friend, sister, aunt.

When a nappy needs to be changed, one of the nurses takes the opportunity to weigh and measure the baby, writing details onto the inside of her wrist.

Inconspicuously she moves to a desk in the corner, takes out an exercise book and enters the figures.

I approach and enquire about the family on the deck. Is this the access visit of the father that she told me about earlier, the one under a Court Order?

'Yes. He's been here a few times now. This is his third week in a row.'

'What's the story?'

'We don't know the details. They just tell us what we're entitled to know, basically just the Court Order.'

'What was the Order?'

'Well, this one is a Supervised Access Order from the Children's Court. It means that the child and the parent can see each other, but only at specified premises – that's ours – and only under acceptable supervision – that's us. Orders like that are generally made for a family with a serious record of harm to a child, or a serious risk of harm.'

The family on the deck is in clear view through the wide windows. Dad is still reading. The nurse can see the entire deck from any place in this large room.

'What sort of harm?'

'Sometimes the child has been taken from the custody of the parent after violence to a child. Or it might not be anything done to the child at all; it could be something done in the child's presence – perhaps harm or abuse to the other parent, sometimes drug taking, perhaps extreme alcohol abuse. Or it could be direct sexual abuse of the child.'

The room and the deck throng with people. They help themselves to morning tea, they bring food and drink to those distant from the kitchenette. Children inside and outside take muesli bars and fruit from low tables. And reject milk in favour of red cordial.

Outside, the father reads on, his daughter leaning close against him, her thumb in her mouth.

22. IN THE ADNYAMATHANHA LANDS

Their eyes mid many wrinkles, their eyes,
Their ancient glittering eyes, are gay.

> (from 'Lapis Lazuli', W B Yeats)

Rocks and trees

For years I have travelled to the Flinders Ranges to work. These are the lands of the Adnyamathanha. White people come here as guests. We are new here. Miners, graziers, explorers, railway men, tourists and administrators – we are new in an old, old land.

Whenever I have the opportunity, I drive the slow route through Angorichina and the Brachina Gorge, where the rock strata tell their story of geological time. At intervals, roadside signs interpret that mute tale. Who could comprehend the antiquity stated?

And, blinded by those honeyed striations glowing in the afternoon light, I have no thought for science or geology. I am a man alone, floored by the beckoning distance, the emptiness and the beauty as the hills fold around me and recede.

It is in the gullies where the water pools deep underground and the great gums grow that I feel the reality of the antiquity of this land and its life. Each tree has individual form and colour and complexion. These vast, vastly old, living things, defiantly robust here in a place of endless heat, speak to me of continuity and endurance. I stand in their silent presence, reverent and small.

Greta and the emu

After driving another hour, I come to the township of Leigh Creek where I am to work. Here I will see Greta again.

Greta is extremely aged, certainly the oldest member of the Nepabunna community. She is the last of a generation that held full knowledge. Her contemporaries were the last completed initiates. When I am with Greta I get that old gum-tree feeling, that same sense of connection with time that has been and has passed.

Greta tells me her stories. She heard these when she was a small girl. My favourite is the story of how the emu lost the power of flight. As Greta recounts her dreaming tale, she smiles that smile, that smile that shimmers light across a room. Her voice crackles with age as she speaks for a while then takes a breather, then resumes. She needs these breaks: her aged lungs and her frail heart are barely holding on.

Greta lives in the hospital now – has done these last several years, going home to Nepabunna for daylight hours only, on birthdays and on Christmas Day. Most days she sits like patience on a monument, awaiting visits from her very many descendants. Thin, frail, pretty in her filmy lilac housecoat, Greta has the presence of one who wears authority lightly. Some of her scapegrace descendants quail before her disapproval.

Greta is engaged with her generations. Although old and now living at a little distance from the clan, she carries the enduring responsibility for children and for children's children, and for their little ones too.

That care for the generations of family sits unevenly in the community. It weighs most heavily upon women; and it is too heavy for some. These lose their gaiety. Passive until moved to rage, these are the mothers with the sad eyes, the fallen face, closed off from joy; enduring an existence that flickers and burns only when re-ignited by passion or alcohol.

Not so with Greta, especially not when she tells her stories.

As Greta tells her emu story, she pauses from time to time to search for a word in English. In the break in her speaking, Greta rests her hand on mine, holding me, holding me in the story, not allowing the dreaming to escape. Greta's hand is long and thin and dry. The skin is pale, almost pink, almost blue, nearly translucent. Her hand sits on mine; I am held, a willing captive.

English is not the language of her childhood. She grew up hearing and speaking Adnyamathanha. English was the new way that they spoke in school. She learned how to speak it well enough for the classroom and for shops and doctors, and she uses it now with her great-grandchildren. They don't have the old language.

The word for emu is *warraita*, but Greta calls the emu *warraiti*. No one else I know refers to the emu that way, but Greta knows what she knows and calls the emu what she has always called her, smiling as she speaks. Perhaps she loves the bird so dearly, she has given her a nickname. Giving a name is always an act of appropriation, of signifying connection.

When I ask Greta if I might write down the story to read to my grandchildren, she is pleased. She wants me to know the story, she wants many, many people to know and understand how the emu lost her power of flight.

Why should she care? What can it mean?

It is clear that for Greta this is no mere story; it is the cause and the purpose of her existence. The telling is an epiphany – it brings her into the realm of the absolute. When Greta recounts the story she removes her shoes from upon her feet, for the land she stands upon is holy; and the bush burns before her and it is not consumed.

Greta has other stories, stories not suitable for ears such as mine. She tells one of these to her friends the nurses.

'There's a bush that grows 'round here, special bush. That one makes things grow, makes them bigger. My sister used that bush. He made her grow.'

'How did she use it?'

'She went out, you know, she take some of that bush, she rub herself, you know – here' (Greta indicates her left breast) 'and here' (Greta passes imaginary shrubbery back and forth across her right breast) – 'and they grow big, real big. My sister – you know her – she come visit me here, she got great big ones. That bush make them grow.'

The nurses are cackling.

Animated, Greta continues, 'And you know Danny? From back home? He use that one too.'

'What did Danny use it for?'

'Well, you know. He take the bush and he rub here' – Greta passes her imagined handful of foliage vigorously back and forth across her pelvis – 'Danny, he grow real big, *real* big – *here!*'

'How do you know, Greta?'

'I don't know. I don't see. But my cousin, she tell me. Danny her boyfriend. She know!'

Greta cannot speak. Breathless, gasping with merriment, she and her friends shake with secret knowledge.

◎◎◎

Year after year, I travel north wondering whether I'll find Greta alive. I didn't come last year and this year, when I arrive, I am too late.

I want to hear about Greta's passing. Whenever I ask, whomever I ask, everyone is keen to tell me. It has quickly become a tale, a community memory of Greta's last weeks and days. Long a legend in the district, Greta herself is passing into myth.

Hospital staff tell me that some roofing tiles came adrift in the hospital and government officials seized the opportunity to close the place down: 'Occupational health and safety are paramount.' Never mind that the problem is confined to a small area, never mind that there are alternative rooms where the ceiling has already been reinforced, the hospital must be closed. Forthwith. Indefinitely.

On the day of the fateful roofing incident, Greta was the hospital's sole patient. Abruptly she was packed up and shipped out to Hawker, 185 kilometres distant, some two hours' drive away.

Lesley was the ambulance driver. Her face creases with sorrow as she tells me, 'They wouldn't let Greta go back to her room to collect her things. I put her into the ambulance and she was sadder than death. She cried. I never saw her cry before. She said, "I will never see my country again."'

Penny was a young nursing cadet at Greta's second home, the hospital in Leigh Creek. She nursed Greta here over some months, and became the old lady's friend. When Penny too was transferred to Hawker, she was shocked to see how Greta had declined in only a few weeks; the gaiety had gone. Penny greeted her friend. No answer; Greta did not recognise her.

Greta's large family came, a carload at a time, to visit her.

They sat, shy and awkward in those cool alien rooms. Greta did not speak. She seemed not to know her own kin.

Penny wheeled her outside onto the deck to enjoy the sunshine but Greta sat, bent forward, cradling her head on her knees, saying something indistinct over and over again. Penny leaned forward to make out Greta's words: 'I want to die. Let me die.' Such words are potent.

Time passed, the hospital in Leigh Creek mouldered unrepaired. The townspeople began to murmur, then to mutter, then were in uproar. A government official appeared suddenly, the ceiling was swiftly repaired and the hospital was reopened.

Seven days before the hospital was reopened, Greta passed away, as one might who had been sung.

Somewhere else

Lyndhurst is situated at the junction of the Strzelecki and Oodnadatta Tracks in the outback of South Australia. These are the map coordinates of the start of the outback; just up the road a bit, the Birdsville Track winds off into realms of white man dreaming. This area attracts mystics and dreamers, hermits and eccentrics – that is to say, people who are not in a hurry.

Lyndhurst sits on an edge: the pub here calls itself 'The Elsewhere Hotel.' It is here that the bitumen roads come to their end and give way to tracts of interminable dust.

Lyndhurst was the best place on the surface of the planet to view the recent eclipse of the sun. This event brought 5000 people to augment, for seven fiery days, Lyndhurst's normal population of around twenty stolid citizens.

Most visitors to Lyndhurst returned home. An exception was the person who was 'treated' in a heat lodge, which is a traditional native American mode of healing. No one knows whether the visitor had an illness to start with. But he was a believer. The believer entered the heat lodge in burning Lyndhurst, and after spending quite some time inside, he was dead – of hyperthermia.

Talc Alf

Cornelius Johan Alferink is a Lyndhurst citizen who lives somewhere else again, in a dwelling a couple of kilometres outside the hamlet. He goes by the name of 'Talc Alf'. Never a person of central tendency, 'Talc Alf' lives on the margin, avoiding the thronging crowds of Lyndhurst's score of souls.

I draw up outside Alf's home and gallery as the day comes to its end. The heat is dying and the place looks deserted. The heat-bleached sand, the dried-out she-oaks, the stillness give me pause. Wondering, stepping tentatively from the car, I look around.

To my right is an open-air gallery where white sculptures sit silently on planking shelves. Ahead of me is a raised area guarded by succulents and other desert plants. Behind this is a structure which appears to be Alf's dwelling, an obscure composite of white stone, mud brick and earth. On my left is a camel yard. The yard has stout wooden rails, a gate, a drum of water – but no camels. Opposite the camel yard is a mechanical contrivance – a couple of metal sails or scoops that whizz in perpetual rotation around a metal pole, which protrudes from the roof of a tubular building of uncertain nature. The sails are flung in their endless chase around the pole by the wind that howls and propels sand in steady streams into my face.

What with the sand and the silent structures that surround me, there is plenty to exercise the eye and the mind while I wait around for signs of life.

Eventually a slow black dog is seen in the gallery. The dog moves in my general direction, followed by a stocky man of middle years. He wears an aged cloth hat and a beard that flows south from the banks of his mouth in waves of grey and white. His face is very pink, while the hat bears an Aboriginal emblem. He wears a look of faint puzzlement. I ask whether I am intruding.

'No, no, not at all.'

I give my name and Alf gives me a soft hand. He shows me around the gallery that showcases his eclectic sculptures, as well as innumerable lapel badges and postcards of the Aboriginal flag. I want to purchase one of these, but Alf won't let me: 'These aren't for sale; just take one, take a few. Spread the word – this is not the country of any queen. This land is Aboriginal land, that's the flag for this country.'

We wander through his gallery and through his Pub with no Beer, a drinkless area of shade. (He has taken 'the Bob Hawke pledge', and has vowed never to drink alcohol again until the Aboriginal emblem is the flag of Australia.)

As we walk, Alf offers comments and histories that are original if not reliable: Did I know? Have I ever wondered? Do I know the derivation of this word, that name, my own name?

Alf is a creative etymologist, who finds origins of words in the myths and mists of cultures and time. He operates with fearless disregard for conventional linguistics, free from the shackles of science and from any narrow academic discipline.

His gallery is peopled with large sculptures in talc or soapstone. They have naturalistic faces and features that merge into universalist symbols, often geometric and recognisably alphabetic. Here and there, names such as Murti Johnny are engraved into the icons. Murti Johnny was an Aboriginal man from this area who was reputed to be the oldest person in Australia when he died aged 114 – 'or so'.

Alf points out a lovely sculpture in milky white talc. It is carved in the form of a woman, beautifully abstracted, with her unborn child. Her form merges with geometric shapes and symbols which Alf interprets for me.

He tells me that this sculpture embodies the story behind the story of Waltzing Matilda. Alf surmises that Matilda was an indigenous woman who carried the child of the jolly swagman. Alf has discovered that the fatal billabong outside Winton is called Combo Creek. He learned that *combo* is the old term for a common law marriage between a white man and an indigenous woman. Alf is certain that Matilda died in childbirth and that the child – a halfblood – was later stolen by the authorities. The swagman could not bear his losses, first of his wife, then of his posterity, so he up and he jumped into that billabong, and his ghost may be heard, as we all know.

'No man,' says Alf, 'would drown himself over a stolen sheep.' He, Alf, knew there had to be a better explanation.

Alf's derivation of this history reveals as much about Alf as about cultural history. Alf is Dutch-born, a boat person who arrived here fifty years ago. He took a wife from Thursday Island.

Alf himself is a combo man. He has a daughter who has recently given birth to a child of her own. The sculpture's soft curves express the tenderness of a father for his child.

We wander into the strange tubular structure beneath the windswept sails. 'Here is my wind-powered washing machine,' says Alf. The overhead sails rotate the metal pole, which is connected by a fanbelt and an old car wheel to his agitator-washer. Inside a paddle wafts idly to and fro, waiting with quiet patience for the consummation of some dirty clothes and soapy water. 'Now watch this,' says Alf, jumping aboard a stationary bike and pedalling furiously. His efforts augment the wind power and the paddle flashes across the inside of the washer and back again in a mighty perturbation of fresh air. 'Now,' says Alf, 'if all the overweight ladies watching too much TV had one of these bike-powered washers at home, they could sit and watch TV and lose weight. Good for the environment, healthy and cheap to run.

'The Pope washing machine people came out here to look at my machine. They seemed very interested indeed. But they left and I never heard from them again ...' Alf is mystified.

Leigh Creek

Thirty kilometres down the road from Lyndhurst is the coalmining town of Leigh Creek. In its heyday, doubtful characters of all sorts gravitated here, and this trend reached a peak when hundreds of labourers arrived to create the new town. Many of the newcomers came with criminal records; some of them were actively wanted in Adelaide. Among them were major villains, others were lesser offenders.

The previous police force of one was an officer well known for his conviviality, a man too much at peace with himself and his parish to handle this later-coming lawless generation.

His successor is a man of unconventional methods. When he arrives in the town, he assembles the entire adult population of

1200 while he reads aloud names from a list of wanted criminals who have drifted here. The police officer names them, then puts aside his list and declares that he knows exactly who is present. He knows but he proposes to forget all about them – until and unless they force him to do otherwise. They hear his warning, he releases them and they keep the peace.

Generations later, Leigh Creek is peopled by white mine workers and their families. They are here for the duration, here until retirement or until exhaustion of the coal or of the expatriate soul.

Copley

A few kilometres closer to Lyndhurst is the hamlet of Copley, which might or might not be named for the ardent practice of copulation here of past years. Here, beside the Quandong Café resides one Tom Agnew, entrepreneur of the copulation industry in this district.

In 1950, Tommy was aboard The Ghan en route to Alice Springs, when it broke down in Copley. He never planned to stay here but he got off, vowing never to take that train again. Fifty-eight years later he is still here. Tall, rangy, scarred by the outback sun, picturesquely earthy in his sibilant Irish speech, Tom Agnew is held by locals to be the improbable heir to a title and estates in Ireland.

Agnew's estate in Copley is distinctive. It is as dusty as Ireland is green. Behind the debilitated structure which is his dwelling extends a graveyard of rusted vehicles. This is Tommy's showroom. His business is the sale of second-hand heavy vehicle parts. If you want a part for your bus or your grader or your 4WD, you'll find it here. Tommy sells to people who do not shop retail.

One of his customers tells me he wanted a part which was nowhere to be seen. Tommy knew where to find it. Bringing out a mattock and a pair of shovels, Tommy had his customer set to work with him, digging behind the corner of his house. Soon, the two struck rust, eventually exhuming the required part. An oily rag removed Tommy's valuable topsoil and the customer left with a part that worked perfectly.

In its heyday, Copley played host to a series of ladies who flew down from Adelaide in the 'fifties to meet the sexual needs of the many single men who worked the mine and who later built the town of Leigh Creek. Nic Klaassen's history, *Leigh Creek, an oasis in the desert*, credits Tommy Agnew with an initiative to establish the copulation industry on a formal basis. He applied to the government for a permit to open a brothel but they knocked him back. So, as Tommy says, 'There were men there desperate for a root; I had taxis in Copley, so I would meet the girls at the airport and book them into the pub, and run men to and from the hotel. I'd be up most of the night …'

As to his own situation, Tommy says, in a voice that whistles and whispers, he's had a number of wives, none of them entirely his own – 'We were never churched, you know.'

The Agnew speech is soft, the elocution an Irish blur. You have to lean forward to hear. The effect is a conversation that feels like a conspiracy. Tommy suspects he has peopled the state with a number of his bastards. He doesn't know for certain. It appears unlikely that his heirs will claim his lands and title in Ireland.

Memorials in Lyndhurst

For a sizable proportion of the population here – both indigenous and non-indigenous – alcohol is a necessary substance. It is needed to silence an insistent sense of cultural loss and estrangement.

In the Elsewhere Hotel in Lyndhurst, the drinkers recall a local who 'got so drunk he decided to do the housework'. Vacuuming his carpet, he initially ignored the dark and sinuous shape he saw on his lounge-room floor. Belatedly the penny dropped and he grabbed his axe and cut the serpent in two. 'Nearly died of electric shock, he did ... cut the electric lead of his vacuum cleaner.'

◉◉◉

Not far away are ochre pits, large deposits of the pigments required throughout Australia for ceremony and corroboree.

People travelled prodigious distances for ochre. Some of these were at war with each other or with the Adnyamathanha, the custodians of this area. Yet through all memory, the Adnyamathanha guaranteed safe passage to outside tribes-people who travelled here for supplies of ochre.

◉◉◉

Outside the community hall in Lyndhurst, truckies and other dedicated drinkers raise a memorial to a late publican who died young while at the wheel of his car. The car disintegrated around him and they needed the Jaws of Life to extract his body from the wreckage.

The deceased was a Mister Alan Dunn. The plaque celebrates 'Dunny – best publican in Australia'. He is remembered for his massive corpulence. He was so gargantuan that he needed to limit his movements to an operating minimum. 'When you finished your drink, Dunny wouldn't give you a refill until everyone else's glass was empty. Then he'd tell you to put all the empties together on the bar, and he'd lean over and fill them all up. Then you'd get another drink.'

The plaque does not mention the blood alcohol level of the deceased publican at the time of his fateful accident. But when the local progress association proposes to name the new community hall after Dunny, Talc Alf raises a lone voice of dissent: 'Aren't we making a hero of a drink-driver? Let's call it the Murti Johnny Hall.'

In the event, the hall bears no name. Only the plaque on a drab stone cairn expresses the fealty to Dunny of truckies who drive up and down the spine of the continent, lonely men of terrible thirst.

And down the road a handmade sign of wood reads 'Johnny Murti's Grave'.

A death

Death calls in various guises. One morning I wander into the hospital to do my rounds. In casualty the curtains are drawn around one of the cubicles. There is no sound, no nurse. I move inside and discover a body on a stretcher. Or is it a body? No human part is visible; from end to end and side to side the form is covered entirely with blankets and towels. Buckled belts secure the inert whole at chest and knee height.

A nurse appears and tells me the story that is not quite a story: 'The ambulance was called to the community early this morning. Someone rang at six; a woman wasn't breathing. A nurse in the community had been doing CPR. When we arrived, the body was warm. The deceased woman lay there in her bed, her husband embracing her. We couldn't see the point in disturbing them with more CPR.'

'What was her medical history?'

'No one knows. Her husband doesn't know. Her kids were standing around, the younger ones crying quietly, the teenagers stunned. We found empty packets of Nurofen-Plus littered around the room. All we know is she had lost a lot of weight; we presume she had a lot of pain.'

I need more information. 'There must be a file here ...'

'No, we've looked. Pika Wiya* don't have any records either.'

We phone the Pika Wiya Service at Port Augusta, but they have nothing.

This woman is a stranger to modern medicine.

I examine the body. No breath, no movement, no heartbeat. The body is cold now, and her pupils do not react to light. She is dead and I certify that fact.

Death has come to an Aboriginal family, coming as it used to do, before science and medical explanations. This is old-fashioned death, mysterious and inscrutable; definite, definitive, implacable; answerable to no one, answering nothing, save for one ultimate question. In its silence, Death silences the fret and chatter of the living.

Before the wailing, a community goes quiet.

Was it a cancer that wasted her body and caused her pain? Or a simple sorrow unnamed that she comforted with codeine? Everyone knows her, but no one knows anything.

A life has ended at forty-three; her husband holds her close as if to hold death at bay; her little ones weep for fear and for loss; while her bigger kids are silent, lacking the language of adults or of children for the grief that will define them.

Fossils and future time

This area has the earliest known fossil record of primitive animals with bilateral symmetry. Once creatures became symmetrical, they began to develop sensory organs at the front end. This was followed very soon – mere aeons later – by a central nervous system. Before too long we had animals with brains, we had thought, purpose, consciousness. We had sculptors and mystics. We had thinkers and drinkers and eclipse gazers. It all started in these lands.

And at some time in the remote past, the Adnymathanha – the Rock or Hill People – appeared with their dreaming. They peopled the landscape, living in a fluid relation to land and time, to plants and animals, to the seasons and the elements.

Now concentrated in the vigorous and contending hamlets of Iga Warta and Nepabunna, where local clans have created cultural tourism enterprises to support their tidy towns, and in Copley and Beltana, the Adnyamathanha are here still.

Nowadays The Ghan bypasses Lyndhurst and Copley and the

tracks are used only by the daily coal train of 115 trucks which snakes south, bearing coal on its way to Portagutta (as some locals pronounce Port Augusta).

Copley coal might well be the lowest grade, highest polluting brown coal in the world. If those facts are not enough to end mining here, the terminal decline in coal reserves will do so in time. When that time comes, the regional hub for services which is the disposable town of Leigh Creek will be dismantled and taken away, leaving unremoved relics to sink like Ozymandias beneath the eternal wind and sands.

Sooner or later, Talc Alf and Tommy Agnew will pass, as Greta has passed. All who came for the coal, and all who adhere to them, will leave.

The guests will go home.

A residual few will haunt Lyndhurst and Copley, custodians of quiet outposts, to service road trains and grey nomads.

But in my vision, the imperishable Adnyamathanha remain in their homelands, just as the emu – *warraiti* – remains; coated in talc and coal dust and ochre and time, they persist.

* Pika Wiya is the name of the regional Aboriginal Health Services in the Flinders Ranges.

23. RUST

Six mornings a week, I get out of bed early and go for a run. Moving slowly on foot through a suburb or a settlement or a city, I catch glimpses of the face of a community and its complexion. Metastasing shopping malls and other scars, beauty spots, sun damage, signs of neglect, tokens of renewal, all show themselves in the light of early morning.

Running through an outback community while its citizens are still asleep, I am seldom solitary. Dogs notice me. Some are curious, some indifferent, almost all are territorial and underfed. These last-mentioned want to join me. They show their teeth, they snarl rather than bark, and they run in packs towards me. I find these dogs unattractive. They make me run faster. They get close enough for me to see their yellow teeth. I pick up a handful of loose gravel and chuck it at the leaders and they lose interest in me.

At work in an outback clinic I meet the regional paediatrician, a blunt and angry man. 'Test the kids' urine,' he barks, 'test it and you'll see they all have protein and blood. They've all got nephritis, all of them.'

I do test urine specimens, and indeed almost all the specimens register those abnormalities, markers of kidney disease. Nephritis is classically a complication of unrecognised or under-treated streptococcal infection.

In Melbourne, post-strep disease is not as common. Doctors kill the streptococcus early with penicillin and the infection remains uncomplicated. But in Aboriginal communities many dogs carry a small mite that causes scabies in their owners. This creates an intense itch. People scratch their itchy bites, creating small breaks in the skin, allowing unseen streptococci into the bites. The sores are so common, recurrent and chronic, the kids so stoical, that many, many cases go untreated. The post-strep nephritis follows. Renal health is permanently compromised and the child usually survives, to be visited in adult years by hypertension and damaged kidneys.

With every positive test I think of that sour paediatrician. The little girls I see skipping rope and playing hopscotch in the school-ground, the boys darting about on the footy oval, leaping, kicking, weaving magic   all of these kids seem kissed by the spark of exuberant life. Can it be true that they carry already the seeds of their early decline into the debility of kidney disease? And all because of their dogs, whether loved or unloved, the intimate companions of their days and nights?

(Only in the Torres Strait communities do I find a systematic program for culling and controlling dogs.)

◎◎◎

Wherever I am I get up early and run. I run because I need to. In Aboriginal communities, when I'm not avoiding dogbite, I have time to notice the deceased motor vehicles that pockmark the landscape. Abandoned by their owners, dead cars are everywhere – in town, out of town, on made roads, on dirt tracks, in the bush – overgrown and shrouded by encroaching scrub. Some stand upright, others lie on their sides. Not only dead, many have been bashed and raped; windscreens shattered, panels stove in, bodies scorched, engines exposed. And rust – rust everywhere.

We Australians love our cars. Whitefellas and blackfellas save up or go into debt for them; we tend them, mend them, wash them till they gleam; buy appliances and optional extras for them, service them and maintain them. We build roads, freeways and garages for them.

We look after our cars better than we care for our health. Cars often live in better houses than outback Aborigines.

As I run in remote communities, it occurs to me that some Aboriginal people treat their cars the way some whitefellas have treated the land.

Over time, I note a mathematical relationship between abandoned cars and community health. The sicker the community, the higher the body count of dead cars. The dead car, destroyed and abandoned, rusts and persists in the public domain, a silent accusation, or confession.

The word that comes to me from history is 'hulks', a name for social shame in eighteenth century England. The hulks, dead ships stuck in tidal mud in river estuaries, teemed with convicts, the people who became the unwilling early population of the colony of New South Wales.

The mathematical ratio of hulks to citizens becomes my predictor of general health, including cultural vitality, alcohol abuse and substance abuse.

In the township of Ngurupai there are few hulks to be seen. One of the few stands like a sentinel on the road from town to the airport – the only made road on Ngurupai.

This vehicle is a truck. I guess its vintage at circa 1950. The lines of this truck please me somehow: a series of cubes and cuboids, yellow duco crusted in rust; a picture of stately decay.

I look at the old truck, the sort of truck I used to see on farms in my childhood in Leeton. Like this old man who jogs past, the truck is in decline. Its slow decomposition seems right, organic. Day after day as I run past it, the rusting old truck speaks to me gently of the passing of time, of universal decay, of the return of all things to our elemental origins.

Through a sequence of ideas, some scarcely related, I muse on an Australian continent in a future time. In a vision of a bleak and terrible future, when some neglect or holocaust of climate has brought human civilisation to an end, that truck, dismembered, collapses into a low heap of rusted scrap metal sitting in the circumambient iron oxide powder.

But the saltwater crocodile survives. In time the scrub recovers. And in the scrub, slipping into and out of sight, another survivor is seen. He is the Australian survivor, *par excellence*. He is the Aborigine.

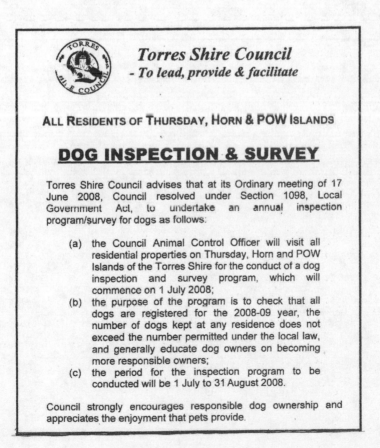

Torres Shire Council
- To lead, provide & facilitate

ALL RESIDENTS OF THURSDAY, HORN & POW ISLANDS

DOG INSPECTION & SURVEY

Torres Shire Council advises that at its Ordinary meeting of 17 June 2008, Council resolved under Section 1098, Local Government Act, to undertake an annual inspection program/survey for dogs as follows:

(a) the Council Animal Control Officer will visit all residential properties on Thursday, Horn and POW Islands of the Torres Shire for the conduct of a dog inspection and survey program, which will commence on 1 July 2008;

(b) the purpose of the program is to check that all dogs are registered for the 2008-09 year, the number of dogs kept at any residence does not exceed the number permitted under the local law, and generally educate dog owners on becoming more responsible owners;

(c) the period for the inspection program to be conducted will be 1 July to 31 August 2008.

Council strongly encourages responsible dog ownership and appreciates the enjoyment that pets provide.

PART FIVE

IN CUSTODY

'The last act is always tragedy. Whatever fine comedy
there may be in the rest of life, we all die alone.

(Herman Wouk, after Pascal, in *This is My God*)

... I emigrated to countries and was questioned by officials and did not understand English. Yes, I would say, yes, yes, yes – because I had fear of the system, coming from Belgium and still having a little bit over from the wartime ...

When I arrived in the US, where I emigrated to when I was eighteen, and you were asked questions: 'Are you a communist?'... I am now talking about 1957 ... 'Yes, I am.' 'Are you here to overthrow the government?' 'Yes, I am.' I didn't understand what I was saying, but I have such a fear of not answering ...

(Magistrate Tony Bloaman who travels to several bush courts in the Kimberley region of Western Australia, speaking on 'The Law Report', ABC Radio National, 21 August 2001)

24. AN APOCRYPHAL TALE?

I mentioned to a knowledgeable friend that I was going to work as a doctor in an outback jail. She asked, 'Which one?'

I told her and she smiled. 'You know, lots of Aboriginal prisoners became healthier there. They got more exercise. They got into a culture of fitness, they spent all their free time in the gym. Later, when those young bucks came out of jail, they were muscled up. Then they went back to their own communities and they scored all the chicks.

'When other young blokes saw what was happening they decided they wanted to get big and strong; then they committed a crime, so *they* could join a gym, as it were. After a while the authorities tumbled to what was happening, so they closed the gym.'

I went to that jail and I worked there, and I checked: no, there was no prisoners' gym.

Later, I raise the subject with my informant. Curiously, she says she's never heard that story, certainly never told it to me – she thinks I've confused her with someone else. No one else has heard the story either.

Perhaps it is apocryphal.

But factual or otherwise, it is in a sense a *true* story; it is a parable in a few sentences that epitomises the tragicomedy of whitefella intervention in Aboriginal health.

25. IN CUSTODY

I press the buzzer and wait for the heavy steel door in front of me to open. Nothing happens; the great door just stands there, grey-green, silent and uncompromising. Now a beep is heard, then a click from the latch, and two jaws of steel gape and release a steel tongue the size of a small tomahawk. I look over my shoulder and farewell the open spaces of beach and sea, then push the door open and pass through. It clunks closed behind me and I stop short before a second door, identical to the first. The process is repeated, the door before me refusing to open until some time after the one behind me is closed and latched.

Between the front door and the clinic I pass through four such doors. None of them will open without a command from an officer in a tower whom I am unable to see but who is able, it seems, to see me. If I want to get to the high security section, the door total will reach eight before I arrive.

I take a step in the direction of the clinic. An officer stops me. 'Did you sign in?'

I do that. The officer stops me again. 'What have you got in the backpack?' I show him my lunch, my notebook, my reading matter.

He is not satisfied. 'Do you have a mobile? An iPod? A memory stick?'

I have all of these; I surrender them to the officer, who locks

them in a drawer. He keeps my driver's licence too. All of my con-
traband is now in custody.

'Don't bring your backpack again, Doctor. Get one of the
regulation carry bags, like this one here.' He shows me a a sturdy
perspex plastic bag.

I offer my hand. 'My name's Howard Goldenberg. What's
yours?'

He grips my hand a little more firmly than necessary, looks me
briefly in the eye, does not smile. 'I'm Officer Mc Gregor.' Perhaps
the officer doesn't have a first name.

This elaborate process of merely getting *into* jail makes me
thoughtful; if it is not easy to get in, it cannot be any easier to get
out. I am a doctor, a contractor here, a free citizen, but I feel a sense
of constriction. How does a person feel from the deep bush or the
coast on first arriving at the jail? Does he realise that he won't sight
the open country or the sea again until he's released? Does he feel
threat or teetering panic?

☺☺☺

The men sit and wait in the yard and enjoy the mild sunshine of
early morning. They are colour-coded, according to the degree of
security in which they abide. The first lot I see are the reds. The
men wear their t-shirts tucked into their dark prison trousers. The
effect, among the plumper ones, is to pronounce the swell of their
tummies. It's a slightly comical look.

No prisoner arrives at the clinic without an escorting officer.
Clad in khaki uniforms of unexpected smartness, the officers are
all a good deal taller than I am, taller than most of the prisoners, powerfully built and of serious mien. They address prisoners
evenly, civilly, without compromising friendliness. They speak the
same way to me. These are disciplined people. They do not wear
firearms. Never have I seen such immaculately polished boots or
such well-suppressed smiles.

Generally the prisoners seem placid. Softly spoken, happy enough to speak to me, most communicate with me effectively. Some, quickly agreeable to anything I ask or request, actually use no words.

After patiently struggling with an unbroken series of densely obscure, almost inaudible responses from this sub-group, I am at a loss. I realise that I need an interpreter. I don't see one.

Come to think of it – for a prisoner group that is more than ninety per cent Aboriginal – there isn't a single Aboriginal health worker. Everywhere in indigenous health, the Aboriginal health worker is the indispensible link between white medicine and black Australia.

Likewise absent are Aboriginal prison officers.

Most prisoners are mature men, mid-twenties to forty years of age, but some are boyish, the odd one as young as eighteen. The young ones, too, seem composed, only the occasional drumming of a hand or the agitation of the legs betraying anxiety.

In the course of what turns out to be a pleasant morning's work, I meet and treat greenshirts, blueshirts and orangeshirts. I introduce myself, ask each person his country, then – because they speak so softly, and because they pronounce the familiar place name with an unfamiliar inflection – I ask again. And a third time. Eventually I get it.

One asks me, 'Where do you come from?'

'Wiradjuri country.'

This bloke doesn't need to ask a second time; recognition is immediate. 'Ah, New South Wales.'

'Yes.'

None of this group of men – and overwhelmingly they are male – has any medical complaint. Almost all look well; they are simply going through the formalities of 'reception' – that's what they call it – into jail.

Here's one, though, who frowns as he walks in quietly and

accepts a seat. He cradles his right wrist which is obviously fractured. It happened yesterday, playing footy. He couldn't sleep last night for the pain. I send him to the hospital for an x-ray and when he returns, his wrist plastered and in a sling, he smiles, his face free of this morning's inwardness.

Here's another, younger man, who has been in only a few days. This fellow is not one whom the nurses call 'frequent flyers'; it is his first time in custody. I ask the questions devised to uncover depression and risk of harm. No, he's not scared, not sad. I show him the Five Faces chart. The faces range from extra smiley, to smiley, through composed, to sad, and deeply sad. The young man points to the middle one.

'Do you have any problems?'

'No.'

'When is your court case?'

'Tomorrow.'

I check his heart and his blood pressure and pulse. They are all okay. He smells slightly of cigarette smoke. I lift his shirt to check his lungs. Beneath the red t-shirt I come across a surgical dressing. Beneath the dressing, a small wound weeps pus. On his right elbow and his left shoulder there are abrasions. The injuries look a few days old.

'What happened?'

'Police punched me ... four, maybe five days ago.'

'Here?'

'No, in the holding cell. I thought my arm would break; they twisted it back, up behind me, real hard.'

'Have you got a lawyer?'

'Yes.'

'Have you told him?'

'No.'

'You should tell the lawyer tomorrow. Show him. It could be important.'

I feel like a conspirator. In the uncurtained, open space of the medical room, I find myself speaking softly, just like my patients do. Do they speak in an undertone because they too are conscious of the ears around them?

I pause, then add the words I would customarily add: 'Tell the lawyer, she can call me as a witness if she needs to.'

Back in the city, a patient responds to words like these as to a gift. Here in this remote northern town, this boy – far from his own smaller community, a stranger to law courts – just looks at me. His face is empty of understanding.

◎◎◎

In the course of my first day I see twenty inmates. All but three are indigenous. It is a day free of menace; free, too, of the demands of the city health consumer. (Only two patients humbug me, both of them white. One wants me to prescribe a special diet on grounds that are no more compelling than a distaste for the prison's mass-cooked food. The diet here is low in fat and refined carbs, healthier than in most homes outside.

My other supplicant, a guest worker from Latin America, wants me to arrange a supply of special vitamins for his eye condition. I know of no eye condition that responds only to vitamins imported from Paraguay.)

◎◎◎

Local newspaper headlines scream: PRISONERS RELEASED FROM JAIL BEFORE COMPLETING SENTENCE.

I read the article and discover that some inmates are released prematurely by a day or two, and only in order to catch infrequent transport back to a remote community. Perhaps headlines like these sell papers.

Around the jail is a fence of razor wire. Until now razor wire is something I have seen only in movies. This fence is about four metres high, over a metre deep, composed of tight spirals of razor hoops. The design is a grotesque geometry – Euclid meets Dali – the fruit of a horrifying mind. Any person who passed through it would emerge as sashimi. At first sight, the scene shocks me. By the end of my term here, I still recoil at its implicit brutality.

After I have completing my term, a senior official connected with the prison informs me that such fencing is outlawed by the Geneva Convention.

Outside the wire perimeter of the jail, two teams are playing footy, eight or ten to a side, in blazing sunshine. The temperature is thirty-five degrees. The footy is of a pretty good standard, good enough to keep me standing a long time in that hot sun. With teams of only eight, the players do a lot of running, punctuated by highly precise passing by hand and foot. The teams are clad in the regrettable stripes of West Coast and – even worse in the eyes of this Magpie supporter – Carlton. I liked the look of these fellows a lot better in their colour-coded prison shirts.

Few of the players are thin. But portly or not, they run, feint, weave and leap like champions. I notice they don't chase much.

I am sorry to report that Carlton wins.

The next day, I treat a second footballer for a fractured wrist and for a couple of fingers that would not have straightened again.

◎◎◎

At the start of the first day, I am disposed to wonder what offence has brought each of my patients to this place of clanging steel doors and murder wire fencing. It feels like an important thing to know if I want to be any sort of holistic doctor. But I don't want my questions to embarrass or shame any of these softly spoken people, especially easy in this open consulting area. I decide that they will tell me if they want me to know. So I hold my peace.

Over the following days some offences are named, most often by the patient who consults me. Many of these people are held on remand, their cases unheard. In this country where one is innocent until proven guilty, these prisoners make no distinction between a charge of, say, assault, and a conviction for that offence. 'I'm in for unlawful entry'; or 'for driving… you know … no licence'; or (almost inaudibly and blushing perceptibly beneath the dark skin) 'for domestic … you know …' The word 'violence' is left unsaid. The sense of shame is eloquent enough.

Similarly in a whisper, an older man says, 'Sexual …' He cannot look at me.

By the end of one day, I have treated two who have killed fellow humans, a multiple rapist, numerous illegal drivers, a few breakers and enterers, one who has injured his wife, one who has done unspoken things to children. All of these deeds were committed under the influence of alcohol, often with other drugs as well.

The next morning, I receive results of their routine pathology tests. It turns out that among my first twenty, there are three syphilitics, two with chlamydia, two with gonorrhoea. Another has hepatitis C. I read the file of the man with hepatitis. The report from his liver specialist amazes me. Initially this man had hepatitis A, B. C and D. Of these only C persists, and this too shows promise of cure.

Every one of these positive pathology reports encodes a story that is hidden from me, stories of shame, of abuse, of ignorance, of stupefaction with drugs or of disinhibition with alcohol.

Hidden stories, hidden diseases, coming to light here, undergoing cure *here* – here in the one place no one wants to be. Recovery and wellness creep up on some prisoners, who will leave healthier than they arrive. Among those who have been inside for a longer time, I see few who are obese and none who is malnourished. Their diabetes and their hypertension are better controlled than elsewhere. They have healthier teeth.

None of the prisoners is aggressive, no one shouts, few appear agitated.

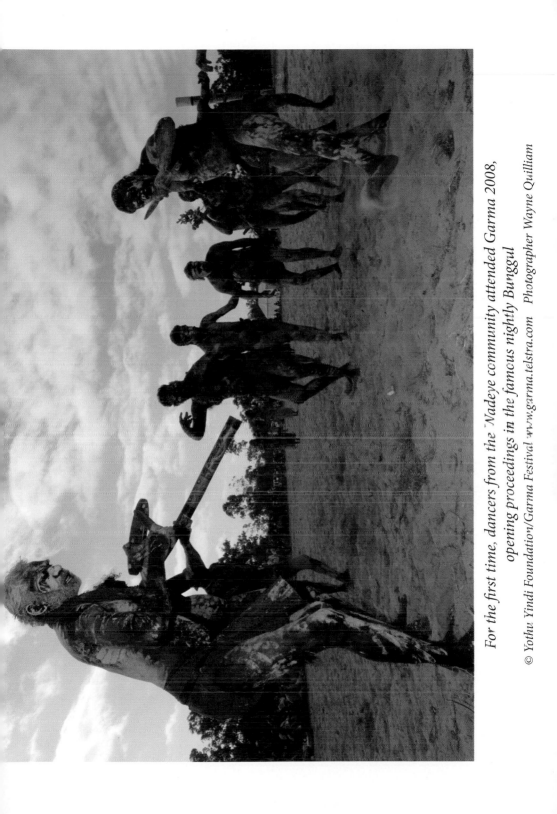

For the first time, dancers from the 'Nadeye community attended Garma 2008, opening proceedings in the famous nightly Bunggul

© *Yothu Yindi Foundation/Garma Festival www.garma.telstra.com   Photographer Wayne Quilliam*

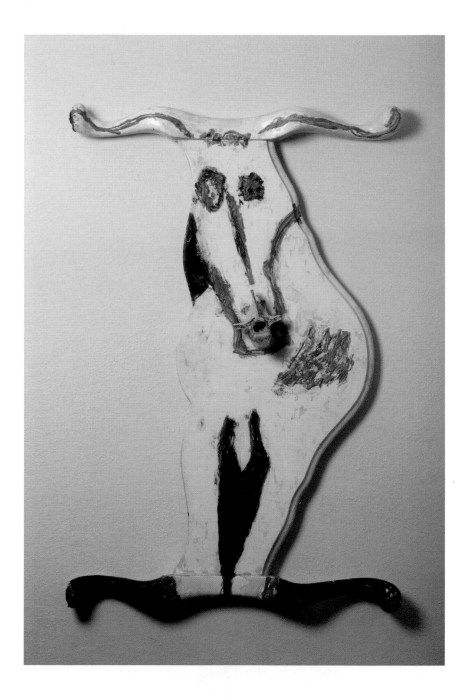

Shaike Snir: 'The White Bull' (p. 208)

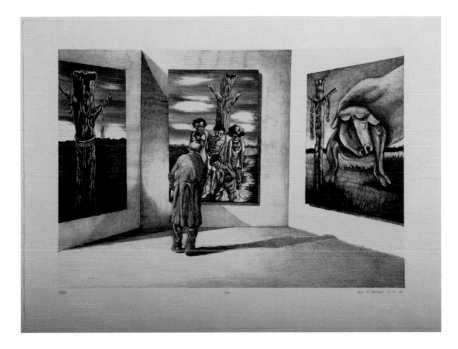

Lithograph by Eolo Paul Bottaro: 'Yosl' showing an aged Yosl Bergner, in caricature, peering at his classic art work from the 1950s which shows Aboriginal people in chains. (pp. 217-18)

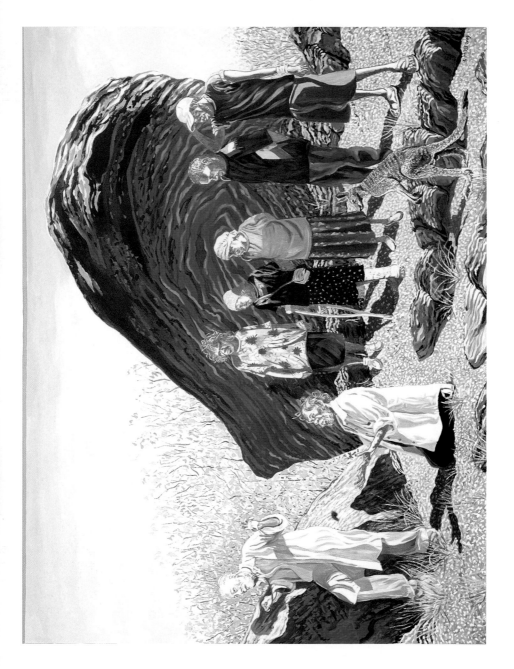

Rod Moss: 'Agony in the Garden: Dr Goldenberg's Diagnosis'

The chief nurse explains, 'That's what happens when humans get three square meals a day, without a lot of fat and a lot of sugar. And consistent medical care … *and no alcohol … and no drugs*.' She pauses. 'Some of our frequent flyers are *glad* to be inside. They tell me, "I am better in jail. No grog here, no ganja. I get better in here."'

☉☉☉

Not all patients are calm. One is an accused drug offender, a white man who just happened to be in the car alongside the 'true' dealer, a Mister Quite Big, to judge by the haul with a street value of $300,000. He is a bit jumpy, his speech hyper-fluent. He wants me to know he is certainly innocent. 'I'll be out tomorrow,' he says. He has already pointed out the injustice of his situation to the police in the following terms: 'If I hitch-hiked and I accepted a ride with a man who had a dead body hidden in the boot, would that make me a murderer?'

Apparently the police officers are not convinced, and when his case comes up the next day, the magistrate is not either. Instead, the court finds the evidence that the prisoner tried to flush cannabis down a watch-house toilet more compelling.

For myself, I sense that his agitation might be the result of abrupt withdrawal from cannabis.

Before I started this job as a doctor in a northern jail, the artist Rod Moss spoke of the people who break into his Alice Springs home from time to time. He knows some of them. 'Mostly, they are kids, just looking for food. They get caught a couple of times and they can go to jail – because they're hungry. Like convicts sent here from their homes in England.'

I tally up my first day's work: twenty patients, almost all of them likeable, with a quiet dignity that belies the ugliness of some of their crimes. The dignified manner, the *humanness* of the perpetrator, does not differ in those who break windows or force locks from those who break or force humans.

By the time I leave jail, I will meet more killers. Fifty per cent of the small group are whitefellas. All but one are thoughtful, highly qualified, civilised humans; the exception is one who is intellectually deficient.

Only the non-indigenous among my patients show any understanding that a trial is an adversarial process, that they might fight, win, even go free. Among the remainder there is a palpable submissiveness. They attend court only to listen, to hear their sentence. Without an interpreter, some will be at a loss to understand even such questions as, 'Are you guilty?'

Out of politeness some will answer, 'Yes.'

◎◎◎

On the second day I meet George. Unlike most of the other prisoners who reside in dry communities and who only come to town to drink, George lives here. He was admitted to the jail yesterday and his case will be heard in a few days' time. He wears a brand-new bandage on the inside of his right wrist.

I ask him, 'What happened?'

'Twelve stitches. A cut.'

'Was it a fight?'

'No.'

'You're left-handed?'

George nods. 'I was mad. It was anger.'

'What were you angry about?'

George looks down, past his large belly, to the floor. After a time he says, 'I haven't seen my kids for three months.' I sense the imminence of tears, but George's eyes are dry.

I ask, 'Are your children far away?'

'No, in town here … but I'm not allowed …' George shakes his head, lifts his injured arm, then drops it heavily to the table top.

I find myself thinking of the man in Melbourne I read about

recently. Following a custody battle, it is alleged that he drove to the top of a high bridge, stopped, got out of his car and threw his small child to her death.

How close was George to that despair? How much safer is he – and his family – with him inside?

George is thinking along similar lines. 'I want some help. This anger …'

In this jail, mental health care is quickly obtained. I meet colleagues here who are experienced and highly skilled. People outside, in our great cities, wait for many weeks for the help that George receives the next day.

◎◎◎

I go in search of Michael, the psychologist, with questions of my own. The nurses are under pressure to convince the doctor to treat a prisoner's chronic diarrhoea. It has been going on for many weeks and it is so severe that the prisoner is incontinent of faeces. His cellmates don't like it. Especially as their fellow inmate doesn't even clean up his mess. He acts as if oblivious of his disgrace. He leaves it everywhere. His cellmates are threatening violence against the defecator if the prison officers don't do something about it.

I study the file. Before admission, Diarrhoea Man suffered a massive drug overdose, ceased breathing, became comatose and was thought to have suffered permanent brain damage. Hence his incontinence, hence his unawareness.

However, later neurological opinion has him fully recovered of his cognition and volition. His anal tone, too, is normal. It's mystifying and it's giving everyone concerned fits of angst.

I ask the psychologist whether he has experience of incontinence in adult prisoners comparable to that of the child who soils himself repeatedly in the classroom. The latter becomes both social victim and perpetrator.

'I've read of it,' says Michael. 'It's adult encopretic behaviour. In an adult prisoner with intact brain function, it's seen as a signal of despair.'

☉☉☉

At the end of the second day the boss's boss, here on a visit from the capital, comes into my room and sits down. After having apologised for being too busy to come and chat with me and to welcome me properly, and then exchanging two-sentence resumés with me, he stops, draws breath and delivers his awful news: 'We discharged a prisoner yesterday, a young bloke. He'd served his term. He went out, got drunk, had a fight with his wife ...' I have a fearful sense that I know what is coming.

'... and he hurt her badly. He was only twenty-two years old. They found him hanging, dead.'

I have many questions. They are too heavy to ask, and any answer will not satisfy. But I wonder which of the Five Happy Faces did that young man indicate, during the process of his final medical assessment?

A paradox: while so many others have died in custody, jail was this man's safe haven.

☉☉☉

On the third day I meet a third killer. He is held elsewhere, on the campus for juvenile offenders. His carers request a visit from the doctor today because his behaviour has changed.

Unlike the adult offenders who are held thirty minutes away, juveniles reside in town. Simple locks and non-razor wire suffice here. A pleasant lady, broad and tall, lets me in. She appears of middle age and when I guess – correctly – that her accent is Dutch, she is amazed; she wonders whether I speak Dutch.

The youth's name is Antony. Gerardina is his prison keeper. She reports, 'Antony's face looked crooked this morning, and he was slurring his speech. And he's been drinking water all day.' Gerardina's own speech has the shushing sibilants of the Dutch

186

English speaker and the homespun phrasing of the adult immigrant. It is pleasant and quite characteristic.

We go to Antony's room. A bulky figure sits on a bed watching TV. He wears navy shorts and nothing else. He has the body of a brown bear and the face of a simpleton.

'Hi, Antony. I'm the doctor.'

No response.

'What are you watching, Antony? Is it any good?'

No answer from my patient.

Gerardina says, 'It's a nature program. Antony loves them, specially snakes.'

Antony's face is unusual. He has the features that doctors used to call mongoloid, that chubbiness, the labrador puppy softness, the cherubic lips of a child with Down's Syndrome. In the centre of Antony's forehead there is a large bony protuberance. It stands fully a centimetre above its surrounds.

Antony is not tall but in his squat corpulence he looks powerful; and in his incomprehension, his simple failure to 'get' what another wants or thinks or fears, Antony is menacing – and innocent of the fact.

I ask Antony some more questions but his semi-syllables of sound do not enlighten me. I examine him; his face is certainly not crooked now, and his facial muscular strength is symmetrical and normal. Perhaps he is over-sedated, or newly diabetic.

A little nervous about the prudence of this procedure, and warning Antony that it will hurt a bit, I stab his fingertip with a glucose test probe. He does not blink. And his blood sugar is normal.

'What medications does he take?'

Gerardina shows me Antony's medications box. He takes tablets for epilepsy – in larger doses than I am used to – and strong tranquillisers. All in all, he takes six tablets each morning and eight at night.

'By the look of it, he'd need to eat them with a knife and fork.'

'Well, no, he doesn't,' says Gerardina. 'He just puts all of them into his mouth at once and swallows them with one gulp. Morning and night.'

'That amount of brain medication would stun a bull. Perhaps we might just ease off on the sedation for about forty-eight hours…'

Gerardina looks worried. 'You don't know what he can be like. Mostly he is a lamb, but sometimes he can be … terrifying. It's taken the specialists a long time to get him right …'

I back off. What are the medical facts here? I see the results before me, but what are the causes? Over and above any chromosomal abnormality, was Antony's brain damaged *in utero* by alcohol or by petrol or glue? Has he acquired additional damage to his brain from his own actions or at the hands of others? Is he a casualty of bush obstetrics – of absent antenatal care, of maternal malnutrition, or of a complicated birth in the bush? Did his brain receive the nourishment it needed in childhood?

Gerardina stands with her back to Antony, and after first ensuring he is engaged once more with his snake show, she speaks softly. 'Antony has had a very difficult life. He was born with brain damage. All the children in his community teased him all the time. Then he developed very bad epileptic fits. When he took a fit, people would stone him, even some of his relatives. He lived a life of misery. Then he got big and strong, and because he does not think well, he's not afraid of anything, and if he gets mad he can hurt himself. Did you notice perhaps, the bump on his forehead? He did that to himself. He was upset, and he banged his head hard – you see he is very strong – he banged and banged against a stone wall. He broke the skin and he splintered the front of his head bone. There was a bloody mush.'

Gerardina's voice expresses the pain of a boy without words, without understanding, without friends. 'And he can hurt other people.' Gerardina pauses, drops her voice further and continues, 'His Mum and Dad were his carers. One day they decided that his tablets weren't doing him any good, and a few days later, he lost his reasoning. He took a knife and he killed his mother. He stabbed his father too, badly, but he survived.

'Then he came to this place. We keep the knives locked away. Antony loves knives. Knives and snakes. His fellow residents don't tease Antony. The boys are terrified of him.'

Gerardina shows me out. There's none of the gaiety in parting that she greeted me with. I thank her and she says, 'All the staff here, we love Antony. We've had him for years … He's nineteen now, too old for this place. Soon he'll have to move to the adult jail, and I'm afraid those people will hurt him.'

As I drive away, I recall Atticus Finch's words to Scout: *Remember it's a sin to kill a mockingbird.*

◎◎◎

On the fourth day, I meet Arnold. He is a well-made man in his mid-twenties with a handsome face. I complete his medical review procedures and tell him he can go. He asks me politely if I have a minute. I do.

Arnold's face is serious: 'I've got an anger problem. I get into fights. I do it all the time.'

'Do you drink much grog?'

'Yes. Not every day, but when I do drink, I drink a lot. I start Wednesday or Thursday and I keep going into the weekend, all through Sunday. That's four or five days a week.'

'Any drugs?'

'Nothing much now. I gave up speed four years ago. Only ganja now.'

(*Only* ganja!) 'Every day?'

'Yes. But not since last month – not since I came in here. Doctor, I've got a good woman. We're having a baby in July – my birthday. I don't want to lose that good woman. I want some help.'

189

Before I prepare a referral for him to see Michael for psychological help, I study Arnold's file.

Entry after entry refers to his risk of self-harm. That good woman could easily lose Arnold.

◎◎◎

The clinic air-conditioning is brutally effective. Dressed for hot weather, I freeze. So I go outside to thaw. I take a seat. On one side are a bunch of women prisoners waiting to return to their cell block. On the other is an officer who will escort them.

Prisoners are speaking in language. The officer interjects with something I don't understand. Apparently his auditors do. They laugh gaily and say something in return. A conversations develops, going to and fro for quite a while. A prisoner asks the officer, 'How do you know Arrernte?'

'I don't. I just speak a bit. I know a little bit from a lot of places.' He says something else and another recognises her language, Pitjantjatjara.

Some more language from the officer and another prisoner laughs with delight to hear her coastal tongue on the officer's lips.

I ask the officer, 'Are you a linguist?'

'No, just a former tour guide. Picked up a bit here, a bit there.'

A bantering conversation resumes. More prisoners join in, names are named, and they ask: does he know this person from Alice, that one from Mutitjulu?

'Yep,' says the officer, 'I know him; and her too. Do you know such and such?'

I wonder whether this bloke will do well in the prison service. Or will they find him too round a peg for this very square hole?

I have questions of my own for the officer. I wait until we are alone to ask them, 'Am I right in sensing that Aboriginal prisoners feel no respect for white man law?'

'Yes and no. It's not a question of disrespect so much as disconnect. Indigenous people feel deeply the claim upon them of "true law", traditional law. White man law doesn't cut deep here. People don't have a spiritual connection to it. They might observe it or they might not. But when the two codes clash, they'll certainly obey traditional law.'

A nurse is sitting outside, smoking and listening in. She adds, 'I know lots of cases of people who are jailed for contempt when a bail hearing clashes with something obligatory, a ceremony or a sorry business. There's an obligation here of kin … they can't not go.'

This is the first of a scattered series of informal conversations I have with prison officers. It is a minority who seem approachable in this way, who show openness when away from their comrades.

On Friday, I am taken to the Bungalows, a misnomer for the dormitory block situated outside the wire. Here reside prisoners of the lowest security. Most will be released in the short term; all have proven good behaviour over time.

As we trudge across the footy ground where Carlton defeated West Coast, I ask the officer whether many prisoners try to escape from the Bungalows.

'Very few. It isn't hard to abscond from here, but very, very few do it.'

'Why?'

'They're not fools. It's not in their interest. They've earned trust by using their brains; they've got privileges here, remission of sentence, very free family access, some go out to town to work or study every day. They aren't going to throw all that away. And then cop an additional term on top of everything else for escaping from custody.'

The officer and I part. As I walk towards my car, the nurse joins me and takes up our theme: 'Anybody'd be a mug to escape from the Bungalows here. What to and what for? You should come here on a weekend; there's family picnics all over the oval, people sneak off for the odd bit of conjugal nookie, someone leaves a little plastic package of something smokeable underneath a rock ...'

26. BLOOD ON THE STONES

I am taking an ordinary *shabbat* walk along the beachside road skirting town, when I notice some red footprints dotting the footpath. The red looks like blood, but it is unlikely to be blood because the iron pigment in blood oxidises rapidly in air and turns rust-coloured.

In other words, though it looks like blood, it can't be that.

Still, they're intriguing, these red footprints that run before me along the concrete path. An adult sneaker on someone's right foot has stepped into something red and sticky and is laying a red sneaker imprint onto the concrete every two metres or so. I think the sneaker is moving at running pace. I also believe there is probably a non-sticky left sneaker moving along at the same pace, without leaving a trace. I guess it's a male footprint, certainly an adult's. (Either that or this is one fast-moving amputee flying along on a crutch.)

This red stuff is really sticky. After two hours of sunlight – for some reason I imagine it was deposited in the dark hours – the stuff remains shiny, a little gooey and thick-looking. Very much like blood.

The bounding steps go on and on along the road, one of the town's longer streets. I follow at a brisk walk; I don't run on *shabbat*. I come to a kerb, cross the asphalt of a side street, climb the opposite kerb, and still the ruddy loper leads me on.

I feel increasingly confident that this is not blood; who would walk or run this far if they were bleeding? (A number of answers offer themselves to that hypothetical question: maybe bloody-foot is not the bleeder, but the bleeder's companion, running for help; or perhaps he is a fugitive from the bleeder. Alternatively, Mister Red Sole could be the bleeder's assailant. But of course it's not blood. These are just the fancies of a weekend stroller with time on his hands and something red underfoot.)

Abruptly the line of footprints comes to a stop. So do I. I look around me and there, just off the path and to my left, is a large patch of the red stuff. It looks like someone has emptied a small-ish can of crimson paint here. Now I get it: a sneaker must have trodden in the red stuff and run fully a kilometre *backwards*, laying red prints, simply to baffle morning comers. Strange behaviour. Really quite odd.

I look up from my musing and note the flashing lights of a police car a few hundred metres ahead of me. The car is parked on the right side of the road which, under ordinary circumstances, is the wrong side. Perhaps these are not ordinary circumstances. Perhaps the blood-looking stuff *is* blood, blood that somehow ignores the rules of oxidation.

Now things make some sense. My man is injured. He bleeds and he runs, runs quite well, with a long even stride and for a decent distance. He is relatively fit or else highly motivated as a person might well be if chased by a blood-drawing malefactor. In which case we might have two fit running types.

My runner, the one I've been tracking, is sober. His gait is dead regular. But where has he gone to? I look down the path in front of me and there, seven metres ahead, the footprints reappear. He must have run two or three paces on the gravel verge after his pause for – for what? – his pause to breathe and bleed?

Now he's running again, but not quite as fast as before. I am following faster. My eyes are down and I'm striding now, entirely absorbed in my bloodhounding, when a voice calls out, 'Get off the path and cross the road! You can't walk here.'

The voice belongs to a police officer who has stepped from her car. Between me and the car, an isosceles triangle of red and white tape encloses an area of footpath and adjacent asphalt.

I stop and cross over, looking backward at a large patch of red sticky stuff on the road, just next to the kerb. Is it my imagination or does that red patch resemble the shape of a recumbent adult human being?

I walk on, my mood no longer playful. Why, I wonder, have I been beguiling myself in fancies this last kilometre or more? Why did I not recognise the bleeding obvious?

I know the answer: I am so far steeped in blood in my day-to-day clinical work in the jail that my mind rebels against more bloodshed, more human violence crashing in and shattering my Sabbath of peace.

An hour later, I walk back pensively. The police car is still there. Forensic types are photographing, taking samples. They label and bag and seal the samples. The one witnesses and countersigns the actions of the other. These deadly serious, seriously proficient young women in police uniform, working in the arena of serious human harm, look incongruously petite and attractive.

I imagine there has been yet another homicide. My mind goes back to the narrative of the very first murder: Cain shrugs … how should he know his brother's whereabouts? Yet the accusation will not be denied: *The bloods of your brother cry out to Me from the earth.*

But as it transpires, the facts on the ground here are darker than mere homicide. The local newspaper carries the following scraps:

> It is alleged that a thirty-seven-year-old woman stabbed a twenty-two-year-old female in the upper thigh after an altercation.

Ambulance officers were able to stop the victim's wound from bleeding. The woman was taken to hospital, where she is in a stable condition.

The alleged offender was arrested and charged with assault causing serious bodily harm.

She was refused bail and will appear in court this week.

◎◎◎

Back at the jail, they ask me to see a middle-aged woman who has a sore neck. She sits hunched forward a little, her thoughts somewhere else, looking subdued. I introduce myself and ask her name. The answer emerges softly through a mouth misshapen and swollen by numerous scars, deep angular gullies, running at angles across her lower face.

The voice says, 'May.' This is a face that used to be shapely and pleasing.

'Is this your first time in here?' (First timers can do it tough.)

'No, four years, a couple years ago. Fighting. I been out a coupla months.'

I ask May where it hurts and she surprises me by pointing to her cranial vault. She shows me a row of steel staples that hold together the edges of a winding rift valley of lacerated skin that has been denuded of hair by a razor. She has more for me to see. She takes my finger in her hand, using it to push aside a hank of curling hair, and points it at another laceration that snakes across another denuded patch at the top of her head. This too is stapled.

Wordlessly, May applies my finger to a further six deep and jagged cuts, all of them long and hairless, every one secured by those disconcertingly non-human hoops of metal. May's scalp is a partially cleared hilltop, with a rail system appearing and disappearing in the scrub.

'What happened?' I ask.

'Fight.'

This seems a massive understatement on the part of the recipient of blows so severe, so perilous, so *heinous*.

'What about your neck?'

'Sore, here.' Once again, my finger is conscripted to demonstrate the locus of harm.

This lady is in pain. But there seems more here than a sore neck and a cut head; May is cast down, sad.

'Do you want to talk about it?' A patently stupid question to ask such a taciturn lady. To my surprise, May does talk.

'It was a fight. I stabbed her.'

I am taken aback. Did I hear correctly? The speech is soft, the tone low, but the articulation and diction are perfect.

May continues, breathing her unhurried confession in a husky undertone: 'She was pregnant. I will be in here a long time; she lost her baby.'

I look searchingly at May, refusing at first to understand. This is no speech in justification or anger: *Not words, but grief, not messages, but sorrow / Hard as the earth, sheer, present as the sea* – a mother speaking, a grandmother, staring as she speaks, at the work of her hands: 'She lost her baby ...' May is giving words to the gravest accusation she knows.

'May, someone attacked you, too.'

No response. Not interested.

I persist, because I must, because I need something to soften that grief in this sorry business. 'May, did she start the fight?'

May nods, then winces, grabs her neck and groans with the movement.

◎◎◎

The hospital released some information to the newspaper, confirming elements of May's story. When the younger woman was admitted near to death from blood loss, doctors thought they could hear the beating of the foetal heart. While intensivists battled to save the mother, surgeons performed an immediate caesarean section. But the baby had died.

◎◎◎

The newspaper carried another story of that Friday night.

> A thirty-eight-year old man was stabbed in both legs with a kitchen knife during an argument. Despite being stabbed in the legs he walked 1.2 kilometres before collapsing on the main road, where, to make matters worse, he was hit by a passing car.
>
> He is in a stable condition in hospital. Police arrested the alleged offender – a fifty-year-old woman – on Saturday morning.

During that Friday night there were two separate knife fights, four persons primed with who knows what intoxicant, armed and fighting with weapons that maim and kill. None of the four was a career criminal, none of those four died; only an innocent, lying in a nearby womb, lost her life.

In every suspicion and supposition, in every deduction, in almost every gender assumption, I was wrong. As Germaine Greer, in her 'On Rage' essay, is wrong. Not all violence is the work of the rampaging male, neutered by history.

PART SIX

JEWISH CONNECTION –
AND DISCONNECTION

For reasons that are often elusive, Jewish and Aboriginal stories spiral around each other, with each turn leading to another unexpected encounter.

Such events always take me by surprise; they are *accidents* in the sense that they play no part in my motivation to go outback. But from the author's name on the cover to the content of these stories, my Jewishness sticks out like my yarmulka.

Initially my specifically Jewish reactions to elements of Aboriginal life surprised me. But it should not have been so. A spiritual attachment to ancestral land that defines the group, the unbreakable bonds of extended family, similar experiences of dispersion, and a history of disenfranchisement, dispossession, humiliation and killings – all these rang tribal bells.

Added to these were accidental collisions with my Jewish self and indigenous ritual, song, story, ceremony; and odd and unexpected moments when remote Aboriginal people recognised my Jewishness and claimed a fellow experience.

Invariably I feel a deeper sense of my Jewish self in the wilderness places where I work. This is the 'psalmist experience', the Wordsworth moment when, surprised by joy, the sentient city visitor comes to a sense of deep rightness in being in this created place. In the outback, any person with a spiritual faculty will experience everyday epiphanies.

While my specifically Jewish feelings have been potent, I think they are fundamentally irrelevant to the universal experience – the ordinary encounter between one self and another. In the long, slow gaze of that encounter, I have seen my own self, unveiled.

27. BROKEN GLASS, WHITE BULL

On 9 November 1938 Heinrich Korn was nine years old.

William Cooper was seventy-seven years old.

Shaike Snir had not yet been born.

Heinrich Korn and his family were proud Germans. Heinrich's father was proud to serve his Kaiser and his Fatherland in World War I. Heinrich (nowadays, Henri) says he only ever began to feel his Jewishness in the autumn of 1938, when he was excluded from his school in Wuppertal-Elberfeld because he was not Aryan. At that moment, the Nazi government created Henri the Jew.

At 11 o'clock on the night of November 9, Henri was awakened by noises from the street. He joined his parents at the window and witnessed unimagined scenes of savagery. Below, by the pagan light of flickering torches, throngs of their fellow citizens, normally reserved and formal people, were cheering and singing wildly.

Heinrich saw uniforms, ordinary householders, gangs of youths. He heard sounds of crashing and the endless splintering of glass. In the moments between the sounds of destruction he could make out some of the singing: *Let the blood flow!*

On all sides in the crowd there was a hideous joy.

From the hallway below them, Heinrich and his parents could feel the thump of approaching booted feet. The footsteps came up the stairs and reached their first-floor landing. Heinrich saw his parents, 'grey with fear'. The footsteps stopped at the Korn threshold. Then they heard a woman's voice ring out, harsh and urgent: 'The Korns are decent people, good Germans, of good character!'

All sound ceased. After long seconds of silence the boots clattered down the stairs.

The voice belonged to their neighbour, Frau Lewitzki, previously no friend to the Korns. Frau Lewitzki had two sons, both members of the SS. It was they who had given their mother forewarning of the 'spontaneous' demonstration. It appeared that neither the local Nazis nor the Lewitzki sons had noticed how similar their Polish surname was to Levi, Levitzki, and other Jewish names.

A friend and classmate of Heinrich Korn, Leo Trosky, died during *Kristallnacht*; when the mob invaded the Trosky flat Leo's parents fought back, the mob seized them and flung them through the window to their death below. Then they took hold of the child and threw him too, to die on the pavement.

Early in the morning of November 10, Henri Korn crept into the street to a scene that 'mere words cannot describe'. Some seventy years later, Henri tells me he cannot speak of it without losing his composure:

> The streets were littered with smashed furniture and thousands of shards of glass … candelabra, brassware, cutlery, bed linen. An upright piano! Dwellings had been ransacked, women were weeping and men were wandering around aimlessly …
>
> One image haunted me: an old grandfather clock, split in two by an axe-wielding maniac.
>
> How strange that we had been spared the horror, thanks to the intervention of Frau Lewitzki. Later I slipped out again. In the city centre, people were in a state of great excitement as the synagogue was burning … I ran towards it with all speed …

A large crowd was milling around, mostly working-class women dressed in their blue aprons, whom I remember as being big and fat. Their faces were twisted with hatred ... they waved their fists, screaming, 'Get rid of the Jews!'

'A woman was attempting to salvage the Torah scrolls and a torch was thrown at her, setting her clothes alight. *People laughed and applauded at a human in flames.*

Suddenly one woman looked down at me and exclaimed, 'This boy is a Jew. I know his face!'

Immediately six heads swivelled and their eyes stared menacingly down at me. I fell on my knees and crawled among the many legs, managing to escape. I was shaking and hid under a bench, ex-pecting to be pursued by an angry mob but nobody came. The burning synagogue must have offered a much greater attraction.

Apparently those efforts to burn the synagogue down failed that afternoon, so the evening brought the experts, who eventually managed to destroy it. The next day, 11 November, I was drawn to see the ruins ... and the gutters of nearby streets were littered with hundreds of torn fragments of Torah scrolls.

For days after, cold and blustery north winds dispersed the Hebrew-inscribed remnants across the city.

Henri stops. He comes back to the quiet and complacent peace of Selwyn Street in Elsternwick. In his beautiful diction, he explains, 'You know we Germans felt utterly abandoned by the world of civi-lised people. Some American Jews – not many – a few twittered in protest. American public opinion was hostile and Jews were cowed. In Britain, Oswald Moseley was describing *Kristallnacht* as "a necessary event", needed to teach Jews a lesson.

'From Australia there was silence. Only William Cooper and his League acted.'

◎◎◎

At the Jewish Holocaust Museum, Henri shows me the plaque that reads:

> The Jewish Holocaust Museum and Research Centre honours
> the Aboriginal people for their action protesting against the
> persecution of Jews by the Nazi Government of Germany in 1938.

Nearby a photograph shows Heinrich Korn embracing a great-nephew of William Cooper.

In Melbourne in 1938, William Cooper read the sketchy reports of *Kristallnacht* in the newspapers and he acted; together with Bill Onus, he organised and lead a protest by the Australian Aborigines League to the German Consulate in Melbourne.

William Cooper was the son of an Aboriginal woman and a white Australian father. He was thus a 'half-caste' in the classification of humans that obtained in his own country and in Germany; he was not good enough to live in the mainstream.

Being of mixed blood, Cooper had to be civilised and Christianised. He was taken from his home to a mission. There he read the Bible and absorbed ideas of the equal value of all humans in the eyes of their Creator. He read too of another people, dispossessed, dispersed and humiliated, and saw his people's experiences in the same light as those of the Jewish people.

This notice appeared in *The Age* on 3 December 1938:

Aborigines' Protest

> At a meeting of the Australian Aborigines' League a resolution was carried protesting against 'the cruel persecution of the Jewish people by the Nazi Government of Germany, and asking that the persecution be brought to an end.'
>
> A deputation of aborigines [sic] will wait on the German Consul on Tuesday at 11:30 a.m., to present the resolution and ask him to convey it to his government.

Cooper's fellow protestor, Bill Onus, was another early Aboriginal activist; his son and grandson went on to become recognised urban Aboriginal artists.

The Onus grandson, Tiriki, works in close collaboration with Shaike Snir, an Israeli-Australian artist, art patron and entrepreneur, eccentric and activist.

Henri Korn and Shaike Snir are contrasting individuals. Henri is a neat man, formal even in his weekend clothes, considered of utterance. He gives birth to his words with careful deliberation from behind the bushes of his Bismarck moustache. His speech is dignified, precise as a physicist's.

Shaike Snir is a picturesque stringbean of a man with the beard of a pre-pubertal billy goat; informal, intimate and intense in utterance, he is a deadly serious joker.

After meeting the Onus family in 1989, Shaike engaged endlessly with indigenous people and causes. His medium and his milieu were those of the artist. In 1995, together with two other Jewish painters, Shaike made a pilgrimage to Mistake Creek in the Kimberley. It was here in the 1930s – in the same historic moment as the massacres of *Kristallnacht* – that a massacre occurred of Aborigines.

A cow belonging to a pastoralist had gone missing; local

tribespeople were suspected; children and women were rounded up and shot.

Later that day the cow wandered back. It was a mistake.

When Shaike arrived he made a gift to the local people. It was an art work of his own making, a white bull, echoing both the cow of the mistake and Picasso's great painting of modern barbarism, 'Guernica'. This was Snir's act of *teshuvah* and *zikharon*, at once contrition and memorial.

He asked Hector Gandalay, a local leader – himself a painter – whether he could forgive the massacre. 'If I do not forgive,' said Gandalay, 'the evil spirit will take me.'

Later, Shaike recruited painters and sculptors from around Australia to contribute to a large-scale touring exhibition on themes of memory and contrition. He called the show 'The White Bull'.

Snir did not rest, did not disengage, creating work after work on the theme of the white bull and the red heifer (an enigmatic sacrifice stipulated in the Old Testament for symbolic penance following sin); and he is working to this day with Tiriki Onus on a major project, recalling Bill Onus and his *Kristallnacht* protest.

As Shaike observes, 'Tiriki and I are good friends. Consider the racial elements: Tiriki is one-quarter Aboriginal. His mother, Jo, is German, so he is half-German. Tiriki is Aboriginal; I am a white man. Tiriki is German; I am Jewish.'

⊚⊚⊚

My nineteen-year-old son is playing pool in a rough pub in inner suburban Melbourne, his customary yarmulka on his head. An Aboriginal man stares at him. At length, the Aboriginal weaves a path towards him and speaks: 'You're a Jew, aren't you?'

Ready for anything, my son replies, 'Yes, I am.'

'Well, us mob gotta learn from you mob.'

'What do you mean?'

'I mean – you mob, you got your land back, you got your culture, you got your pride ...

'We gotta be like that.'

AFTERWORD

WANDERING IN DOTHAN

I have been writing and publishing stories of my encounters with Aboriginal Australia for some time. Since 1990 I have spent numerous periods, each of a couple of weeks or so, working as a relieving doctor in remote places. A fortnight is a laughably brief time; continuity is one of the most valuable aspects of a local doctor's care, and in indigenous communities a doctor is not trusted quickly. By these standards, my mercurial visits would be of no value. But a fortnight allows some respite to a doctor who does make a difference. Such is the scarcity of doctors in the bush that I am invariably invited to return to the community.

Some questions arise: what am I, a white, middle-aged, middle-class person doing, writing in other people's backyards? It's true that Aboriginal people have suffered loss of lands, independence and culture. Is it not a further dispossession that a stranger takes it upon himself to tell their stories?

The simple answer is: I need to tell stories in order to make sense of my life. All I can do is write what I see.

What is it I am looking for?

As usual a suggestive answer comes to me from Bible stories. The answer is the one that Cain is unable to give in reply to the question: 'Where is your brother?' It is the answer that the young Joseph gives to a mysterious stranger on the way to Dothan (read 'the outback'). Joseph is a favoured younger child, born into privilege, the darling of his father. At his father's behest, he sets out to 'see the peace' of his brothers. Wandering, lost, he encounters the stranger who asks, in a suggestive future tense, 'What will you seek?' Joseph's reply: 'It is my brothers whom I seek.' I too recognise that need to be close to my brothers, both those of my blood and those of my land.

What have I found?

Aboriginal Australians are not at peace. They are unwell, underfed, overfed, afflicted excessively by our lifestyle diseases, confused by our drugs and drink, endowed with income but not with work, living in sickening poverty in paradisiacal places; and distracted from their serious cultural business by the trappings of our serious cultural emptiness.

I have found Aboriginal people gentle, harsh, patient as the earth, sudden in anger, explosive into fraternal violence, hilariously humorous, outgoing, shy, culturally bereft and culturally rich beyond our ability to dream. I have heard (but not personally seen) innumerable stories of abuse of power or trust on the part of empowered persons, stories of the most painful betrayal.

With every encounter I have found fresh contrarieties; this list will never be complete. I have found complexity that needs to be acknowledged before it can be addressed; depths that must be respected; and I have developed a splenetic distaste for simple solutions. Invariably these seem reductive, simplistic and insulting.

I have found myself uncomfortable in many ways. I have felt helpless, and confused by my helplessness; irrelevant and occasionally absurd. I have experienced shock and moral disorientation. Numb hopelessness followed, then a phase of toxic resignation. Later came a calmer state of acceptance, which left me open to encouragement; and mostly now I maintain a poised refusal of acceptance.

I go to where I do not speak the language, either literally or metaphorically; places where I am on the wrong foot culturally and socially. And in medicine, where my own community accords me some secure status, I am here often at a loss. My patients' understandings of health and my own are not congruent. Nor are they precisely opposite, but elusive and quite literally secret.

I struggle to reconcile my notions with theirs. Without such a reconciliation, without translation from human to human, we are two persons, unequal and uncertain, standing on shifting sands with power moving constantly between a potent prescriber who has the power of words and a patient wielding the power of silence.

At times, within that groping uncertainty, I am lost, looking for my brother. I witness scenes that distress even veteran workers in these communities. In Mutitjulu once, I met a nurse who said, 'I'm leaving, my time is up.'

I wondered whether she had completed a contract.

'No,' she said, 'You know when your time is up.'

'How do you know?'

She looked away, fell into a silence, then replied, 'The horror. You can't take any more of the horror.'

Gazing into that heart of darkness, I too have felt my composed self fray and start to unravel. And so I write these stories which are my own. But there are rules, constraints and safeguards that I create and observe.

The stories are true but the names of people are not. (There are two exceptions, both of whom are public figures. They are quoted as they speak to me outside of a clinical setting, where medical confidentiality does not apply.)

I have rendered some place names opaque. These measures are intended to protect privacy and should spare a bereaved reader the pain of coming across the name of a deceased person. In a number of instances, I have fused, divided or grafted one half of a true story or one part of a true person onto another. The result is a story about a created person. The person's true identity is a secret. But the story, I warrant, is true.

AUTHOR'S NOTE

Those are pearls that were her eyes (p. 19) is from Shakespeare's 'The Tempest' (I ii).

No motion has she now ... (p. 19) is from 'A Slumber Did My Spirit Seal' by William Wordsworth.

'After Uluru' first appeared in *The Age*, A2, August 4, 2007. Subsequently it appeared also in Australianreader.com

A version of 'After Uluru' appeared in *Wet Ink* (Issue 10, Autumn 2008) as 'There's Been a death ... '

Sections of 'Next Door to Paradise' first appeared in the November 2008 edition of *Cyclamens and Swords Publishing* online magazine.

The lone and level sands stretch far away (p. 147) is from 'Ozymandias' by Percy Bysshe Shelley.

The bloods of your brother ... (p. 195) is from Genesis 4:10.

The lines *Not words, but grief ...* (p. 197) are from Les Murray's 'An Absolutely Ordinary Rainbow' (*The Vernacular Republic, Poems 1961-1981*, Angus and Robertson, 1982).

ACKNOWLEDGMENTS

In the course of my work and of the writing of this book, I have been a guest in Aboriginal communities on about fifty occasions. I thank my hosts for their hospitality and for their tolerance.

In late 1938, a group of Kooris protested to the German Consulate in Melbourne against the Nazi atrocity that was *Kristallnacht*. Their action did not succeed in altering the history of Europe. Instead, it set a high-water mark in Australia's concern for the unfortunate Other. It made Australia a better place, and for this act of unprovoked kindness, I acknowledge and thank my Koori brothers.

Raft might have sunk before its launching without the support of very numerous friends who read chapters and gave advice and suggestions. Among these, it was Martin Flanagan who insisted I publish these stories in my own voice; and Helen Garner who urged me strenuously to publish the pieces she liked and to incinerate those sections – 'posturing and rhetorical' – that she did not.

Colin Hockley, Maria Tumarkin and Irene Hayes were invariably tactful; Neville Stern, Lionel Lubitz, Sally Bird, Steven Leslie, Robert Hillman and Nick Miller were kind enough to object to the objectionable and condemn the contemptible. My particular thanks go to Irene Hayes, an endlessly willing literary archaeologist.

My daughters, with their uncanny eye for a father's errors, have directed that eye with candour to the text of *Raft*, to its great benefit.

Sue Blashki introduced me to the Koori Children's Court and helped me to excise inaccuracies in matters of procedure. Likewise, Natalie Seigel showed me how the procedural tragi-comedy unfolds as the blackfella faces a whitefella court of law.

Rod Moss is a Ferntree Gully boy whose eyes were opened when he moved to the Centre twenty-five years ago. He was the first to open my eyes – through his art, his written word and his lived friendships – to the backyard of my country and to the peoples who live there. I thank Rod for permission to use his painting 'Raft' on the front cover, and 'Agony In The Garden: Dr Goldenberg's Diagnosis' on the back cover.

Shaike Snir contributed his art works, his high ideals and his abiding quirkiness in the preparation of this book.

Thanks to Eolo Paul Bottaro for permission to reproduce the lithograph 'Yosl' showing an aged Yosl Bergner, in caricature, peering at his classic art work from the 1950s which shows Aboriginal people in chains. The panel on the artist's left is of Bergner's very recent work, titled 'And the Chains Remain'. The third panel visits the 'White Bull' theme of Shaike Snir's own work (referred to on p. 208) and his exhibition at the Geelong Gallery.

I salute Brendan Finn for the mastery and subtlety of his photography that revealed the artworks in their beauty.

My editor Anna Rosner Blay deploys a remarkable array of indispensible gifts – a keen eye for the ugly phrase, the tact of a diplomat, an obsessive drive to double-check references and quotations; and a respectful reticence in her approach to the delicate ego of a writer.

My publisher Louis de Vries loves books and writing and authors more than he loves money. No writer deserves a publisher like Louis.

When the material for a book is gathered in the course of dozens of absences from home, the writer becomes an absentee husband, son, father, brother, *Saba*, doctor, colleague and friend. I thank those whose goodwill I presumed upon, those who forgave me and those who did not.

My son Raphael, like all my children, was kind and helpful in rescuing a hapless father from his inattention to life's realities. He also acted as my legal guardian.

Finally to Annette, whose dignity and constancy have sustained the fabric of a family; whose love brings me home, who *is* my home.

> So long as men can breathe or eyes can see,
> So long lives this and this gives life to thee.
>
> (Sonnet XVIII, William Shakespeare)

Howard Goldenberg
Melbourne May 2009

A SHORT ANNOTATED BIBLIOGRAPHY

Bird, Carmel: *The Stolen Children – Their Stories* (Random House, 1998). A small book of long sorrowful sighs.

Flanagan, Martin: read any of his writings for one man's relentless quest for meaning as a non-indigenous Australian. Flanagan explores the great Australian religious enterprise – the practice of sport – to trace expressions of the spirit. Again and again, he considers the life and sporting practice of the indigenous athlete to illuminate the broad experience of being Australian. Subtle and thoughtful writing. Not simplistic.

Greer, Germaine: 'Rage', Melbourne University Press, 2008. Greer derives her confident understandings of indigenous violence from her study of a vast array of scholarly material. It is striking to read such clear diagnoses made at such a distance. Apart from a couple of apparently brief visits to outback communities, Greer's ideas seem to be based on scholarship and her own intuition. Forthright and simplistic.

McMillan, Andrew: *An Intruder's Guide to East Arnhem Land* (Niblock Publishing, 2007, 2008). This unsentimental, unflinching, witty, uneven work on how intruders raped Arnhem Land won the Northern Territory Book of the Year Award in 2008.

Moss, Rodney: artist and writer. Visit his web page at www.rodmoss.com to see how a mainstream painter coopts and adapts indigenous modes of painting to themes from classic European traditions. Read anything he writes, but especially, 'Funeral at Santa Teresa'. The catalogue of his show 'Even As We Speak' is available through the Uber Gallery website.

Also for an analysis of Rod's work read the article 'Rod Moss' Royal Portraits' in The Bureau of Ideas at www.thebureauofideas.com/texts/sep2003.pdf

Rothwell, Nicolas: a poetic and prolific writer on Aboriginal art and culture in Northern Australia. He has a nose for the mystical, the ancient, the threatened and the doomed; and an unmatched, intimate acquaintance with innumerable elders, law men and artists.

I find enlightening his writing about indigenous artists, and thought-provoking his stance on intervention and recent policy initiatives.

Siegel, Natalie: a young lawyer from Victoria. Google her for illuminating reports on Aboriginal disadvantage and entanglement in whitefella law.

Note especially a transcript from Radio National's Law Report on Bush Courts (below); and read 'Bush court: administering criminal court process and corrective services in remote aboriginal communities', a paper presented at the Crime Prevention Conference convened by the Australian Institute of Criminology and the Crime Prevention Branch, Commonwealth Attorney General's Department, and held in Sydney, 12-13 September 2002 (www.aic.gov.au/conferences/crimpre/siegel.html)

Snir, Shaike: Israeli-born, Melbourne-based painter, art dealer, idealist and busybody. For insights into his singular crossover between art and activism, and for its lineal connection with the great Australian-Israeli artist, Yosl Bergner, see the Geelong Gallery catalogue accompanying the exhibit 'Return of the White Bull' (21 February-12 April 2004)

The Law Report: Bush Courts – Part Two, 21 August 2001, www.abc.net.au/rn/talks/lawrpt/stories/s349743.htm

An enlightening series of conversations between Damien Carrick of the ABC and a number of persons with close experience of Bush Courts in the Top End and elsewhere.

Trudgeon, Richard: *Why Warriors Lie Down and Die*, published by Aboriginal Resources and Development Services Inc., available from Openbook Publishers, GPO Box 1368, Adelaide, SA, 5000; and from ARDS, 191 Stuart Hwy, Parap, NT, 0820.

This is the single most enlightening book I have read on causes and cures for indigenous 'passivity'. If you want to grasp the essential complexity of indigenous Australia, read Trudgeon.

To find out more before you purchase, visit www.ards.com.au, choose Why Warriors from the side bar and open Executive Summary.

Also by Howard Goldenberg

My Father's Compass

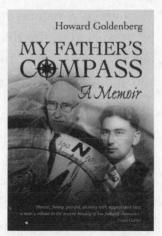

"A delicate, unflinching, profoundly loving portrait of a very complex man." *Helen Garner*

"Howard Goldenberg is a fine wordsmith and a wonderful storyteller. He explores his father's life with great compassion and honesty. His compass has served him well both as a doctor and a writer." *Paul Jennings*

"I thoroughly enjoyed this book and the real emotion it delivers. Howard is a natural story teller. The reader drifts from lines that will make them laugh out loud about childhood exploits, quite seamlessly to the compassion parent and child can have for each other in the beginning, middle and end of life …

This moving Australian story is peppered with a generous insight into the Jewish culture as well as a little poetry. It is a rare treat. If readers have been hesitant to pick up a memoir until now, then this is the perfect introduction." *Deanna Smith, ABC Brisbane*

"How can a faithful Jew, a man described through his long life as observing the commandments, refuse to believe in anything he was told without seeing the evidence for himself? Yet this is the conundrum which permeates Howard Goldenberg's beautiful and painful biography of his astonishing father. Howard, a Melbourne doctor, spent more than 57 years observing his father, Myer, in the most minute and intimate detail, and the result of such intimacy enabled him to write a beautiful memoir, *My Father's Compass* … a delightful and complex exploration studied with wit, passion and luminous respect." *Alan Gold*

"Howard is a natural storyteller and it is through his numerous light-hearted stories that we gain insight into his father's religious faith and personality. An unusual memoir and tribute by a sensitive son, guided by his father's compass." *Lionel Sharpe*

"*My Father's Compass: A Memoir* is eminently readable, replete with family vignettes and mostly amusing anecdotal recollections, and lends itself either to being devoured at one sitting or, if you are the kiss-and-run reading type, being sampled and digested in installments … One of the most endearing qualities of *My Father's Compass* is the tongue-in-cheek style …" *Jerusalem Post*

Howard Goldenberg grew up in the Riverina town of Leeton, New South Wales. On his father's side, Howard is descended from the Gaon (Genius) of Vilna; on his mother's from Cyril Coleman, pearl diver, polo player, and one-stringed violinist, of Broome.

He practises medicine in both city and outback communities.

Howard is married, with three children and five grandchildren.

In 2007 he won both the Victorian Country Marathon and Northern Territory Marathon Championships (over 60 years) and is currently training for his thirty-seventh marathon.

Raft is his second book.